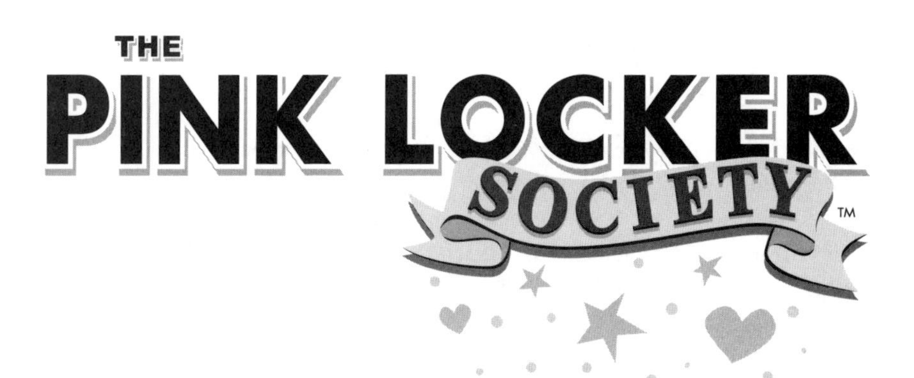

Debra Moffitt

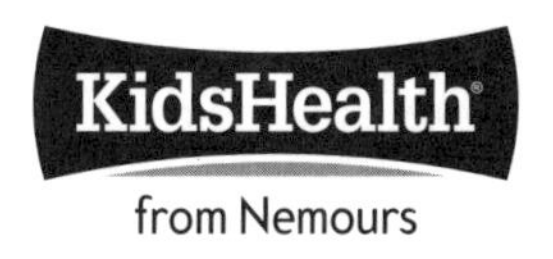

The Pink Locker Society™ is a KidsHealth® book written by
Debra Moffitt and published by Nemours.

Illustrations by Chuck Gonzales. Cover design by Matthew J. Luxich.

The middle school name, "Margaret Simon Middle School,"
is used as a tribute to, and with the permission of,
Judy Blume, author of *Are You There God? It's Me, Margaret.*

PinkLockerSociety.org

Educators and librarians: for a variety of teaching tools,
visit www.KidsHealth.org/classroom

Library of Congress Control Number: 2008938594

ISBN 978-0-615-23826-5

Printed in the United States of America
December 2008

First Edition

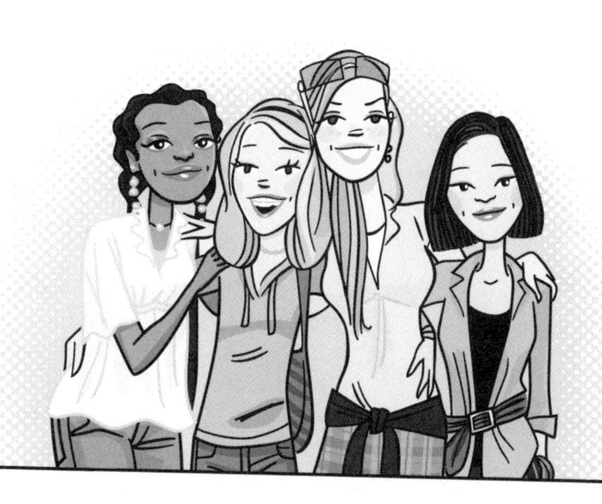

A big thanks to all the curious girls
who visit KidsHealth.org. Your
no-nonsense questions, lively
opinions, and heartfelt stories
inspired me to write this book!

THE PINK LOCKER SOCIETY™

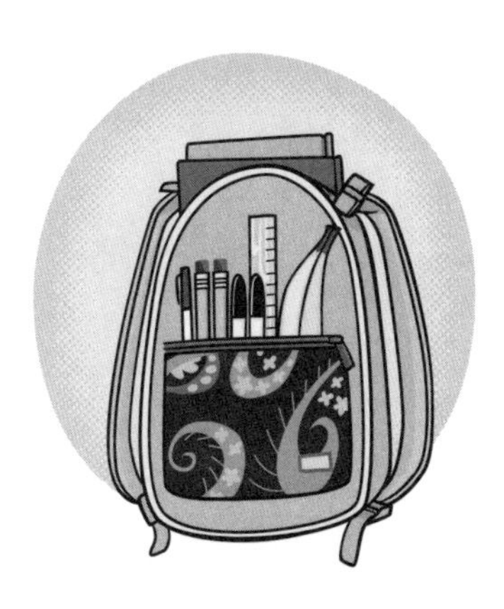

Chapter 1

For one and only one day of the school year, I am so excited that my body works as its own alarm clock. Waaaaaaaay early in the morning, my eyes pop open. I wake up to my quiet room, my cat purring on top of the covers and sun streaking through the window. My clothes are clean and ready, waiting for me on a hanger on my bedroom doorknob. Socks are tucked inside the shoes I'll wear. My lunch is in the fridge and my backpack is loaded with new pens, pencils, folders, and even a few "supplies" in case my you-know-what shows up at school.

My body alarm turns off – way off – for all 179 school days that will follow this one. On those days, my bed holds me down like a magnet and I simply can't-can't-can't move. And I don't move until my mom calls me for the third time, when her voice gets that "Jemma, I'm not foolin' around here" sound. But today, she doesn't have to call at all. I'm not tired. I'm wired. I could run a marathon or bake a cake before the bus comes. Energy runs through my arteries and veins and sparks up and down each strand of my wavy blonde hair. I want 8th grade to start and start now.

BEEP! I dig through my already-packed backpack for my phone. It's

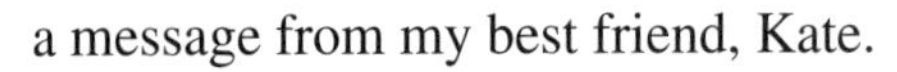

a message from my best friend, Kate.

KATE: Forrest alert!

(That means she's already on the bus and she's spotted HIM. Forrest McCann.)

ME: wearing?

KATE: camo shorts w/ blue t

ME: sigh…

Who wouldn't want 8th grade to start right away? Eighth is what I call one of the "royal" grades. There are three of them. (Four, if you count kindergarten, which is its own kind of royalty.) The core royal grades are 5th grade, 8th grade, and 12th grade. Get the connection? Royal grades are when you're in the top grade at your school. In other words, you get to be queens (and kings) and rule the school that year. The top-top-tippy top would be 12th grade – the senior year of high school with the prom and driving cars and all of that. But 8th is magic, too.

Ask an old person (like a parent, for instance), and they'll probably say there's not much difference between the first day of 6th grade and the first day of 8th. OK, it is true that any 6th grade girl at my school, Margaret Simon Middle, will…

1. Eat breakfast.
2. Get dressed.
3. Fix her hair.
4. Grab her backpack.
5. Hop on the bus.
6. Look for her friends.
7. Go to homeroom.
8. Open her new locker and move in.

9. Hope for the best.

But look more closely and you'll see these two first days are as different as Alaska and Hawaii. I should know. I've visited both – the states and the grades. The 6th grader doesn't yet know that at Margaret Simon, headbands are in and barrettes are out. She doesn't know that you need to pick a spot *beforehand* to meet your friends or you'll never find them in the crowded lobby.

Our 6GG (6th grade girl) doesn't know to sling her backpack over only one shoulder. And unless she's what my mother calls an "early bloomer," she doesn't know that over both shoulders she needs a B-R-A. Even if you're Flatty McFlat Chest, like me, you still wear a bra. It's part of the uniform.

The 6GG will fumble and fuss with her new locker, which is way bigger than the one she had in elementary school. The lockers at Margaret Simon are seafoam green on the outside, big enough to stand up in, and the combination lock is built into the door, like a bank safe. So there our girl will stand, clutching a damp slip of paper with the combination written on it, backpack hanging from both shoulders, and two pancakes flying free under her shirt. The locker won't open on the first try, or the second, making the first day of 6th grade feel as bone-cold and lonely as Prospect Creek, Alaska, before sunrise.

But if you're in 8th grade, like me, you know the rules of the school. Today, a hot and steamy August morning, my headband was in place. The bra was on board. My backpack was hooked to only one shoulder. My two best friends and I had already decided to meet where we always do – at the water fountain near the auditorium doors. In fact, we had even specified that if that area was too crowded (or if Taylor Mayweather was doing one her MSTV broadcasts there), we'd meet next to the vending machine instead.

And when it came to my locker, no sweat. I calmly headed to the number they assigned me (2121) in the 8th grade locker block. I approached my new home, already armed with a little shelf to make the space more workable, a mirror so I could check my teeth for food particles after lunch, the photos I wanted to stick on the door, and even tape to get them stuck. I spun the dial of the combination lock, feeling as tropical and sunny as it was outside. I could have danced the hula after I heard the "chunka-chunk" that told me I hit every number of the combination just right. And on the first try, too. Aloha, 8th grade!

But that's where this story gets kind of funny. Not "someone dropped their tray in the cafeteria" funny, but funny-strange. My mother once told me that there are certain days that you just know are going to change your life. Like, the day you start college or the day you get married. From that point on, she said, you know lots and lots of stuff is going to change. And you'll have this new dividing line in your life – with everything that happened before being on one side and everything new on the other. My mom is always saying stuff like this. (If your mother is also a poet, you know what I mean.)

"Don't worry," I told Mom, "I can't go to college for another five years and nobody has asked me to marry them." (This was almost true.)

"And," she said, "there are other days that are just as life-changing, but you don't see them coming. Life can surprise you."

Today was one of those days.

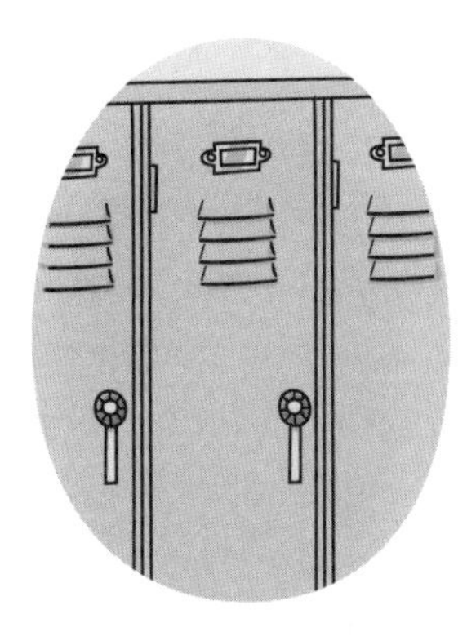

Chapter 2

OK. I didn't hula dance in front of my locker, but I did swing the door wide open in a ta-dah! kind of way. I almost whacked Clementine Caritas, my locker neighbor to the left.

"Jeez!" she said, blocking the door with her perfect hand, tipped with perfectly shiny red fingernails.

"Oops. Sorry! Don't know my own strength."

Tall as a tree, Clementine was not a friend. As she looked down at me, I studied her face as everyone did. She was a genuine teen model and had photo shoots in New York, Los Angeles, and on funny little islands that I'd never heard of. Clem wasn't pretty in the blonde and fluffy way that Taylor Mayweather was. Her face was all big gray eyes and angles – a high and wide forehead, strong nose, and jutting cheekbones.

As awkward as it was nearly bashing the precious head of a teen model, I was glad my locker door didn't swing open the other way. If it did, I might have hit Forrest, the kind of guy you cannot stop staring at. That he was my locker neighbor to the right was another reason to hula, at least mentally. A whole year of opportunities to say "hi" to the hottest guy in school. Did I mention he was Taylor Mayweather's boyfriend? Or that I had known him since preschool? Seriously! When we were 4, we used to be partners and had to hold hands all the time.

My new locker let out a breath of cool air and I stood for a minute to enjoy its emptiness, like a brand new apartment all my own. So many possibilities. My mind was on all the organizing and arranging I wanted to do. But before I could reach for my tape, something shined at me from where the back wall should have been. It was the door to another locker.

This one was hot pink and glossy. Attached to the pink door was a note:

Shhh!
You are now a member of the Pink Locker Society.
More details to come.
Shhhhh!

Remember that stuff about the dividing line? Draw mine here.
I inhaled a short, sharp breath, dropped my armload of books, and slammed the door. I even thought about leaning against it the way they do in cartoons. Was somebody in there? Was I supposed to open that pink door? Was this a joke? All my stuff lay in a heap while everyone else busied themselves with interior locker design.

Clem looked at me coolly. If she wasn't such an ice princess, I might have pulled her down to my height and showed the inside of my locker. Instead, I decided to say, "I'm fine." Trouble was, I couldn't even say that. After my gasp, the words stayed locked in my throat. As for Forrest, he didn't notice me (big surprise) or my gasp. I tore around the block of lockers, looking for someone I could tell.

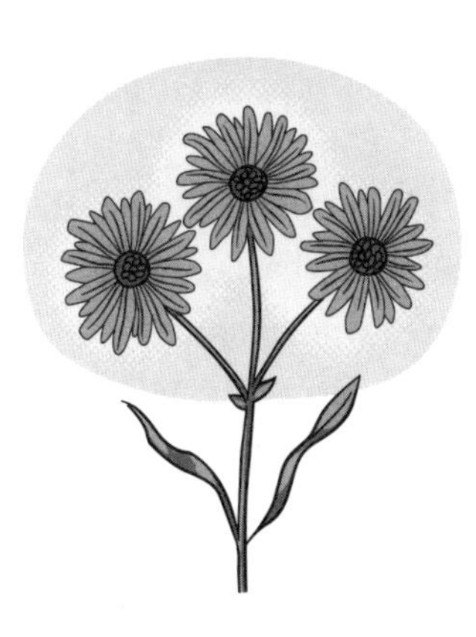

Chapter 3

No surprise who I was looking for: Kate (BFF1) and Piper (BFF2). I turned left once, and since everyone still had their heads in their lockers, I starting scanning the backs of heads for Piper's auburn ponytail and Kate's brown braid. Nothing. I turned the next corner and found them both. They were standing close together, almost touching, as they stared into a locker. They looked like they were studying a painting at the art museum.

"Guys!" I said, a little out of breath. But they only made eye contact with me for an instant before turning back to the locker.

"I just…(pant), found something crazy in (pant) my locker."

This time, they looked up and locked eyes with me. They said nothing but they parted so I could step in between. We bunched close, the three of us, like flowers on the same stem. All six eyes saw the same thing: a glossy pink locker door. Same note, too.

I felt hot and drowsy, the way I did before a test, or when Forrest brushed by me. I looked around and saw no one else standing in amazement. Some were still taping and stacking, but most seemed to be finished with their locker work and were beginning to wander toward the

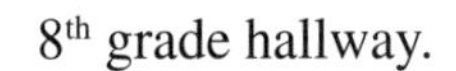

8th grade hallway.

"There's one in Kate's locker, too," Piper said. "I'm opening mine."

"No way!" I said, pulling her back by her shoulder. "It says 'more details to come.' We have to wait."

"Shhh!" Kate said, then whispered, "It says 'Shhhh!' too."

"It does *not* say 'do not open'," Piper said, "so I'm opening it."

Piper crossed in front of me, stood sideways, and reached one bare arm into her locker. She looked like she was feeling for something under a bed. I heard her tug on the metal latch, but it wouldn't open.

"It's locked," Piper said.

"No duh. It's a lock-er," Kate said. "You need the combination."

Piper stuck her head way inside the locker, popped back out again and said, "This lock has letters on it instead of numbers."

Just as I was about to have a look for myself, the bell rang for first period. People scattered. Piper shrugged and Kate walked toward her locker. I rounded the corner and saw my stuff in a heap, like a building that had just been torn down. I quickly turned the combination lock on my regular locker. Chunka-chunk. It opened. Without looking, I threw my stuff inside and went to class.

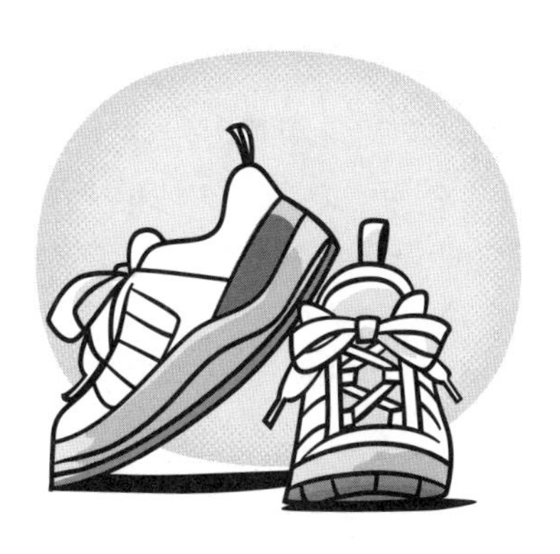

Chapter 4

For a few days, we didn't know what to do. Piper kept tugging on the pink locker door, but it was always locked. Kate did an Internet search on the Pink Locker Society and found something in the university's archives. Trouble was, you needed a password to see it. And me, well, I pretty much tried to avoid my own locker. When I did have to open it, I acted like there was a hungry beast asleep inside. I was very quiet and pulled my books out very gently. I closed the door firmly, but never slammed it.

Aside from the pink locker, 8th grade wasn't starting out all that magically. I didn't understand geometry, Forrest had not said so much as "hi," despite 13 locker encounters, and I still hadn't gotten my you-know-what. On the bright side, the new gym teacher was nice and said, after we ran a lap, that I should consider going out for track.

Did you know aloha means more than one thing? It's hello, goodbye, and a whole bunch other stuff. It's even a technical term that has to do with sending radio and satellite messages. So what did I mean when I said "aloha" to 8th grade?" I meant hello, bring it on, let's chow down at the buffet of exciting times in store for me, Jemma, an 8th grader.

Eighth grade was my chance (finally!) to be popular. Not Taylor Mayweather or Forrest McCann popular – and definitely not as popular as Clementine Caritas. But I did want the easy-peasy grade 8 popularity that just about every 8th grader gets to have. We are owed it. But how popular can you be when you're me – the only girl in 8th grade who's afraid of her locker?

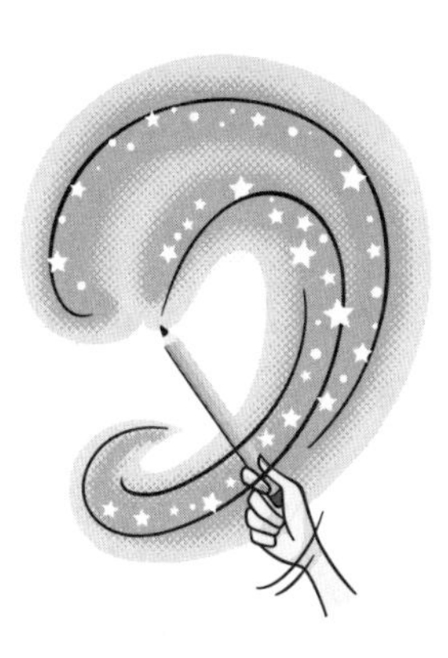

Chapter 5

On Thursday, the "Shhh!" note was replaced by a new one. Of course, I didn't know because I hardly ever stopped long enough to look in my locker. But Piper and Kate spotted their notes and, sure enough, the same one was stuck to my pink locker. I had been too spazzy before to notice the pretty pink stationary and the fancy way the letters were written, like a wedding invitation. This one said:

First meeting of the Pink Locker Society
Friday at 1:35 p.m.
To open your pink locker, use the following letter combination:
S-E-R-V-E
This combination will be activated ***only*** *from 1:35 p.m. to 1:36 p.m.*
The meeting begins 5 minutes after the start of the study hall period. You have been excused from this study hall.
Enter through your ***own*** *pink locker door! If too many girls are climbing through the same locker, it attracts attention.*

We looked at each other, back to the locker, and at each other again.

"We are going to go *through* the locker door? Through to where?" I asked.

Nobody answered, but Piper smiled wide. "This is unbelievably cool. It's like Larry Potter or something."

"*Harry* Potter. And Margaret Simon isn't Hogwarts," said Kate. "We're *normal* girls. It's not like we can do magic or something."

"Not yet…" Piper said, flicking her pencil at me like a magic wand.

I grabbed her pencil and gave her an exasperated look. "Nobody is doing any magic. I don't know about you guys, but I'm not going in there tomorrow. Notice how it doesn't say anything about when the meeting is *over*."

Kate pointed out that the note said we were excused from study hall, so we'd be out at 2:10 for our next class. Sometimes she was cautious like me, but not this time. She was going. And Piper, of course, couldn't be stopped.

"I'm not saying I'm not nervous, but I think you should go," Kate said. "It really is an honor."

"What do you know about it, Kate?" I said. "We don't even know what the Pink Locker Society is."

"I know a little," Kate said. "I know that it's good. That's all I can say.

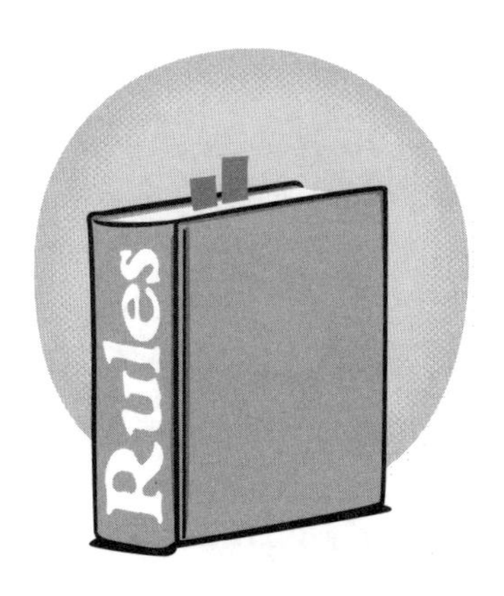

Chapter 6

Did you ever have a friend who always reads the instructions on the inside of the board game box? I don't mean she reads them to figure out how to play. I mean she already knows how to play but she reads the directions to improve her grasp of each little rule. If you're not properly spinning the spinner or discarding your cards the right way or adding up how much the bank owes you, that girl will let you know. That girl is me.

Piper could care less what the real rules are. And Kate falls somewhere in the middle, which is good because she keeps Piper and me from having a jillion arguments. Unlike Piper, I liked rules, needed them even, and so far there were no rules for the Pink Locker Society. Which was probably why I was having so much trouble with all this. That night, on the phone, I tried to squeeze out more information from Kate about the PLS, but she wasn't talking.

"Just show up tomorrow at 1:35," she said. "I'm bringing my camera."

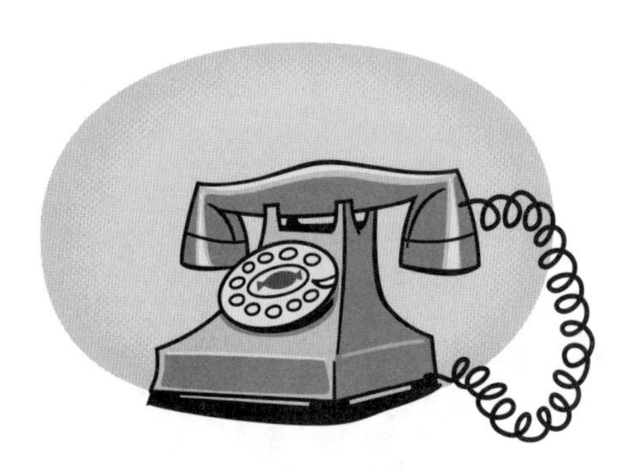

Chapter 7

For the first time in recorded history, the school day went fast. Too fast. Before I knew it, I had finished lunch and we were just one period away from the Pink Locker Society meeting. I really wanted to know how we had been excused from study hall. What if it wasn't true? Did I really want to get detention for skipping class? Although, technically, study hall wasn't class – or was it? I'd have to check the school handbook on that.

Math flew by like it's never flown before. I never thought I'd ache for another parabola, but I was disappointed when Mr. Ford said that was all for today. He told us to use our first study hall of the year wisely.

"How you spend your daily study hall can very well determine the course of your entire school year," he said.

You don't know how right you are, I thought.

I stopped in the girls' bathroom after class and waited until 1:33, giving myself a minute to get to my locker and a minute (why did we have only a minute?) to use that funky letters-instead-of-numbers combination. S-E-R-V-E. Serve who? Or as Mom would say, "Serve whom?"

The 8th grade locker block was exactly that – a big square of lockers. Piper, Kate, and I were on three different sides. My locker was in the middle on the east side, facing the bathrooms; Piper's was in the middle of west side, near the windows; and Kate's was in the middle of north side, near the stairwell. In the long days until today, we wondered if that meant something. If you had looked at it from an aerial photo, we formed a sort of triangle.

At 1:34, I stood in front of my locker almost alone. Everyone else had moved along to study hall. I pretended to be looking for something until the last straggler left. My face felt funny – quivery – as I examined the combination lock. The alphabet circled the dial.

1:35! I took the dial between my thumb and pointer finger and started spelling. S-E-…This was harder than I thought. Once I put my head in the locker, it blocked most of the light. I found R….now where was V? Earlier, I did the math to determine how many seconds I had per letter – 12. I thought that was more than enough, but it wasn't when the clock was ticking. Suddenly, I had big floppy clown hands and I couldn't see. Finally, I found the V. Now on to E…

Ugh! I went past it! Now, I have to start over. Breathe, I said, don't panic. S-E-R…I heard voices from behind my pink locker door – the other girls were already in….

"Miss Colwin," a voice called from the real locker side of the world. It was Mr. Ford.

"Is everything all right?"

I spun around blocking his view of the pink door.

"I'm fine. Good. Great. Thanks. Just looking for something. Going to get a jump on that extra credit you just gave out."

"OK," he said. "Then off to study hall with you, Jemma."

"Sure. Will do. Thanks."

I turned around and waited for the sound of him walking away. The pink locker remained shut. I had to start over again and it was now too late. 1:37. Ugh! I had missed my chance. I tried the combination again, but the locker wouldn't budge. I sat down, my back to the pink, and wondered what to do next. I was angry at myself, but relieved I didn't have to go in, and worried about (and maybe jealous of) my friends.

When doors (of any kind) opened, why did they always go in and I always stayed behind? I pulled out my class schedule and tried to see where my study hall room was. But the computer-generated schedule was no help. Instead of a room number, it said ***. I couldn't go to study hall even if I wanted to. I was a woman without a country.

At least I was until I heard some noise from inside my locker. I also heard voices as I jumped up. A moment later, Kate opened the pink locker door. It swung in instead of out and she pulled me in by my forearm.

She whisper-yelled to me, "Watch the step, watch the step!" but it was too late. It was one of those steps that's three or four inches steeper than it should be and throws you off completely. I was in, but I was down on one knee, like I was waiting for someone to say, "On your mark, get set, go!"

Kate pulled me up, reached in to close my real locker door, then closed the pink one. Her camera was hanging on a strap around her neck and I was very glad she hadn't thought to take a photo of me at this particular moment.

Piper helped me up and said, "Have a nice trip?"

I usually say, "I'll be back next fall," but my brain was too busy drinking it all in. First of all, my knee hardly hurt because I had fallen onto a soft rose-colored carpet with fringe on the ends. We were in what looked like a super-rich old lady's house. There was a living room area filled with formal furniture, needle-pointed pillows, lamps with glass domes over them, and lace doilies on the tables. But big sections of the rest of the room were closed off by thick, plastic tarps. The place was clearly under construction and there was a fine coating of dust on a long table where 12 people could have sat comfortably for dinner.

A large, boxy pink telephone sat in the center of the table. The earpiece was attached to the phone with a twisty cord, and instead of push buttons, it had a spinny thing, like the phones in old movies. The phone was tethered to a big silver speaker.

Oddly, on the dusty table, someone had left us snacks – fresh fruit salad and a glass pitcher of lemonade. Music was playing, something old with lots of horns (duh-nuh-nuh-duh-nuh-*nyah!*). The woman singing was spelling something, but I was too distracted to figure out what it was. A short flight of wood stairs led to a loft, where I could see desks with machines on top of them. Were they sewing machines? I should've worn my glasses.

"I hope they're going to renovate the bathroom next because it could use an update," Piper told us, pointing over her shoulder at a closed door. Her mother was a real estate agent so she knew a lot about the finer things in bathrooms these days, like granite countertops, dual showers, and soaking tubs. "Very vintage stuff in there. But at least the toilet works."

"I told you this was good," Kate said, pinching my arm.

I thought about how people say "pinch me" when they're dreaming. Kate pinched me and I didn't wake up. We were at school, somehow inside the block of 8th grade lockers, in a secret room. It was a huge space, big enough to live in. There was even a little kitchen, also mostly hidden behind a dusty plastic tarp. But aside from the construction work, it was hard to feel at home. Who lived here? Who might come strolling down from the loft?

Kate spun around and said, "You should know we have company."

I heard water splashing on the other side of the closed door. Then it opened and a girl I never saw before stepped out. She was tiny, perfectly put together, and her shiny, black hair was gathered in a pink bow at the nape of her neck.

"So sorry. I guess I was nervous. It was…quite an urgent matter," the girl said, speaking perfect English, too perfect to have learned the language in the United States.

"I'm Bet," she said. "It's a nickname. It means 'duck' in my country."

"Bet is from Thailand," Piper said. "Her family just moved here this year."

Bet and I said hello, and then there was so much to say that no one said anything for a while. We dug into the fruit salad, poured lemonade, and talked mostly about what we were snacking on.

"Good cantaloupe" was all I could contribute.

After a while, Bet pointed out her locker door. On this side of the world, it had her name written on it, like a movie star's door: Bet Hirujadanpholdoi.

I wanted to turn around and see mine, but the phone on the meeting table rang. Bet let out a squeaky squeal and her hands flew up to her face.

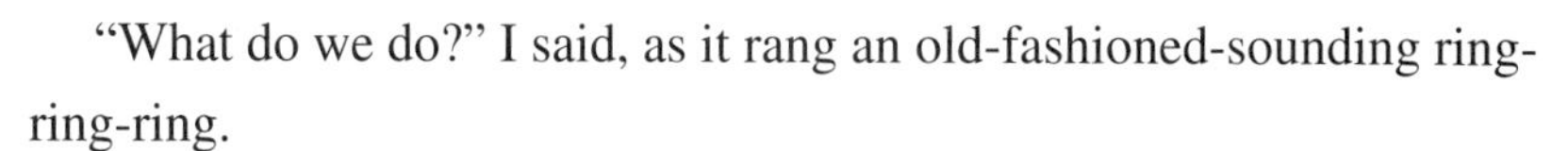

"What do we do?" I said, as it rang an old-fashioned-sounding ring-ring-ring.

"Pick up," Piper said.

"Pick up, but be polite," Kate added.

I picked up the pink earpiece and said hello.

"Hello, dear!" a kindly woman's voice called out. "Can you hear me OK? Flick the silver switch on the phone, please."

I snapped the silver toggle to the right and the woman's voice filled the room. The sound quality was scratchy, like when you're ordering something from a drive-thru. She sounded a little like my great-aunt Agnes.

"Let me first say welcome – welcome to you girls. I know this is a little disorienting. Believe me, I know. But this is going to be an important day for all of you!"

She went on to say we four had been selected by "members emeritus" of the Pink Locker Society, formerly the Pink Locker Ladies. This secret organization was dedicated to serving the girls of Margaret Simon Middle School – and had been since 1958, she said.

Whoa. We were shocked. A secret society operating in our boring school? I wanted to know more, much more. Like, who were last year's society members? They would be in high school now, but at least we could ask them what was up with all of this. But when I asked about last year's group, the woman on the other end of the phone didn't answer.

"Well, there was a…an unfortunate interruption in our history. Can you hold on a minute?"

Before we could say yes, we heard the woman murmuring to someone else. It seemed like a long time before she got back on the line.

"Well, where were we? You girls have been selected to restart our chapter. This has been years in the making!" she said.

Seeing as though we didn't know what she was talking about, we didn't know what to do next. Should we applaud, yell "hurray!" or just keep quiet in the hope that she would start making sense? The four of us stayed silent.

"Does anyone here know about the PLS?" the woman asked.

Kate raised her hand, like she expected to be called on.

"Anyone?" called the voice on the phone, unable to see Kate's raised hand.

I nudged Kate and she said, "Me."

"That must be Kate," said the voice.

"Kate has been selected for the PLS through one of our most interesting channels. She is what we call a 'legacy' – someone in her family was a Pinky! And now Kate can carry on the noble tradition."

"What the heck does that mean?" Piper asked, her mouth full of grapes.

"Of course, of course, you want to know," the woman said. "The PLS serves middle-school girls in need. We have a network of members both current – which means you four – and past – which means women your mothers' age and older. It's a vast network to support you in your work."

Piper looked at me the same way she looked at me earlier today when our English teacher wrote "iambic pentameter" on the board. Kate pursed her lips like she does when she's trying to keep a secret. I gave her a "What gives?" sort of look, but she said nothing.

"What is this 'work' of which you speak?" Bet asked in a small voice.

"Sorry, dear. I didn't quite catch that," the voice said.

"I think we – I mean, everyone but Kate – is still a little confused," I told the phone voice.

"Oh, yes, of course!" the woman said. "So little to say, so much time. I mean… reverse that. The Pink Locker Ladies – I mean the Pink Locker Society – performs a valuable service here at Margaret Simon. Any girl who has a problem or question can get it answered quickly, accurately, and with the kindness we have built our history upon!"

Kate stayed quiet, but Piper and I kept asking away.

"What kind of questions?" Piper asked.

"That's what you're going to find out once they start writing in. In my day, it was a lot about growing into a woman – changing bodies and so forth. Some things change, but I suspect that as long as there are girls, they will want to know about PBBs."

Even Kate was mystified.

"PBBs?"

"Oh, sorry, dear. That's periods, bras, and boys. Nothing draws a crowd of girls better than those topics."

Piper laughed out loud and Bet's hands flew to her face again. Kate shot me a look and smiled. PBBs were the topics we discussed 99% of the time. But none of us, except maybe Piper, would have considered herself an expert.

"How are we going to help them? Take appointments like a doctor?" Piper asked. "I would look really good in a white doctor's coat."

"Oh, no, dear. We give advice confidentially. Back in the day, girls would drop off their questions in little wooden boxes hidden around the school. But today, I'm proud to announce, we're launching PinkLockerSociety.com! They can send in their questions from the website and you'll post the answers."

"What if we give the wrong advice?" I asked.

"Oh, you won't, dear," she said.

I wasn't convinced. If someone or some book had all the answers about PBBs, I would be happy to learn, I thought. But before we could ask who or where we'd find such a thing, the voice said, "Check your mailboxes on the way out. You already have your first client for the year. Good luck and think pink!"

The question on the tip of my tongue was this: How could I, who knows almost nothing about PBBs, give advice about them? In fact, I could give advice only about one B – bras. And even that was limited to what my mom told me as I tried on the available "training bras" at Blume's Fine Kiddie Clothing.

I had a few other questions for the phone voice, if you'd like to know: Who was she, this grandmotherly woman who never told us her name? How were we going to run a website? Why were we picked for this job? Who brought the snacks? And who was that singing over the stereo speakers? I really liked her big voice and the chorus was really catchy. She was definitely spelling something (R-E- something, something).

When the speakerphone fell silent, Bet was the first to speak.

"Do you imagine we are getting graded on this?"

Piper and Kate both laughed, but I didn't know if Bet was serious or making a joke. I'm still not sure. And who was Bet? I had never seen her before – and neither had anyone else. I wondered if she would be hanging out with us now. We were the Gleeful Threeful, as my mom always called us. Get it? A *three*-ful. It had been that way ever since we were toddlers. Our moms met at Yoga Baby class and we'd been entwined like pretzels ever since.

"I am so totally jazzed about this," Piper said, spinning around in a high-backed chair at the conference table. "I feel like a business typhoon in here!"

"It's tycoon," Kate said. "Typhoons are bad storms." Piper was always reaching for a word and picking the wrong one.

"What are we supposed to do now?" I asked.

Before Kate could answer, we heard the bell ring. It was 2:10, the end of study hall. Instantly, pink lanterns I hadn't noticed before switched on. They were posted above our locker doors, like torches to light our way. Our individual doors were located in the middle of each of the huge room's four walls. I thought we formed a triangle, like a mysterious pyramid, but with Bet, we were just a big square. On this side, the locker door was the same hot pink, but it looked more like the front door of a house.

"Call me tonight!" Kate called as we split up to go back through our lockers. Before I opened the pink door, I grabbed a thick stack of papers from the "mailbox" – a plastic pocket at my locker door. It was sort of like the mailboxes I'd seen in the teachers' lounge. Then I took a big step up, carefully clearing the step I fell down on the way in.

The inside of my locker was dark. And I wondered how I would pop out of it unnoticed. Inside, I waited for the sounds of people walking past to fade away. Then I slowly pulled up on the inside latch, light spilled in, and I stepped back into the real world.

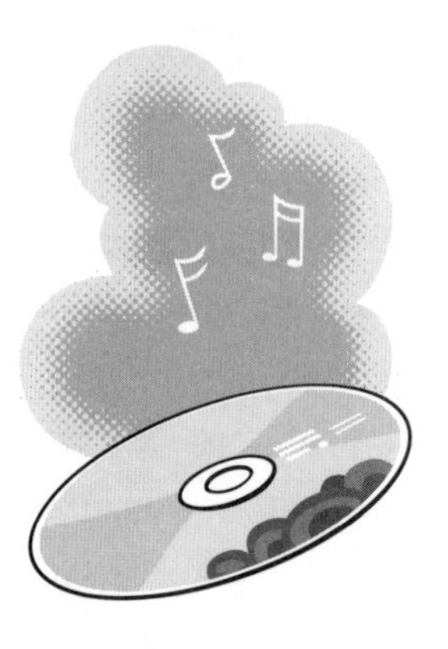

Chapter 8

On the bus ride home, I sat alone and started reading my PLS mail. Actually, I devoured it, looking for more information that would make this picture come into focus for me. Even though I knew more than I did on the first day of school, I was still pretty fuzzy. There was some helpful stuff in my stack of mail, including a short history of the PLS.

There was a calendar that included our regular meetings (every school day during study hall) and the word combination for each day. Next up was R-E-S-P-E-C-T, which sounded oddly familiar. The packet also included an entire pad of hall passes in case our work took us out of the office during study hall. (Cool!) And there was a key labeled "elevator" (?!). Then I came to a file of papers about our first assignment. The report said our first "client" was a 6th grade girl, identified only as M.G., who submitted the following question:

Dear PLS,

I'm in 6th grade and my best friend already has her period. I want mine, but also sort of don't. I need to know **exactly** *when it will come. It needs to come soon and not at school for the first time. Please help! I*

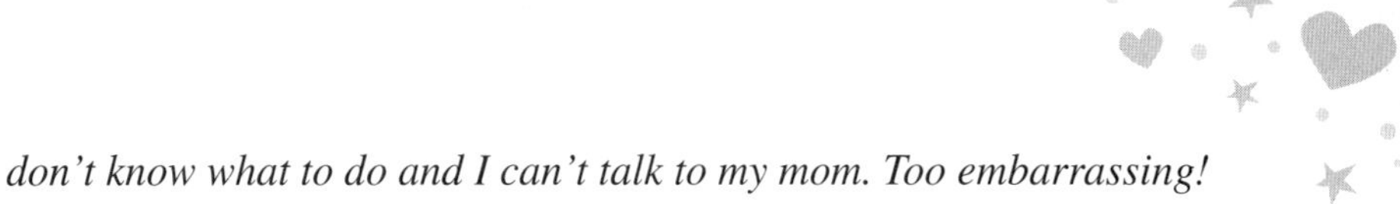

don't know what to do and I can't talk to my mom. Too embarrassing!

Your friend,

M.G.

The question hit me like an ice cream headache. Just when I was starting to think I might like this Pink Locker Society stuff, POW! Here I was, an 8th grader, and not only did I not have the answers to M.G.'s question, I, myself, was still waiting for *my* period. I couldn't imagine sitting around that big conference table in the PLS office, admitting to Piper and Bet that I didn't have my period and dreaming up some answer for the 6GG.

I was pretty sure I was the only 8th grader who had this problem, but only Kate knew I was still waiting. Piper always assumed that I had mine. She even once asked me for a pad because she forgot hers. Luckily, I always keep them with me, just in case. But before I could get too deep into M.G.'s question or think much about my situation, I read an instruction in bold type on the title page of the file. *STOP. Do NOT answer any client's question until you have read the PLS Rule Book.* I leafed through my thick bundle of mail and fished out a slim gray book. It looked used, like something you'd find in your grandma's attic. But finally, here were the rules. They began on the first inside page.

Failure to read and follow each of these rules will result in immediate dismissal!

At this point, I wasn't sure I even wanted to be in the Pink Locker Society and this was telling me how easy it would be to get kicked out. Still, the handbook was a happy discovery. Here's what it said on page 4:

1. *Enter the PLS office only during study hall – 5 minutes after the final bell.*
2. *Give high-quality advice. Don't guess. Learn and share your knowledge.*
3. *If you don't know how to answer a question, use the PLS-SOS system. (See Volume II.)*
4. *The PLS is a secret organization. Do not talk about your work or give the pink locker combination to* ***anyone*** *under* ***any*** *circumstances.*
5. *The PLS is not a clique. To honor our history of grace and hospitality, be a friend to all.*

Some of the rules I understood completely. Others I half understood. And a few left me completely clueless. A PLS-SOS? I was also confused by the pink CD tucked inside the pages of my handbook. At first I thought it might be electronic files, but it was a little more retro.

When I put it in my laptop, it started playing music – the same music that was playing in the PLS office. But retro or not, the music was good. Turns out that confident-sounding singer was someone called Aretha Franklin. And the word she was spelling was indeed familiar. It was R-E-S-P-E-C-T.

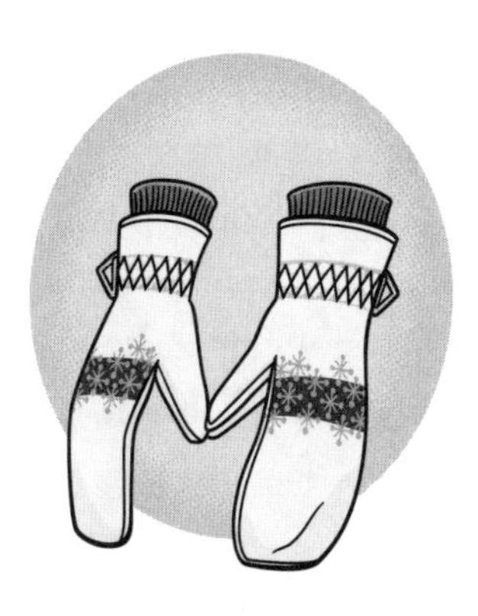

Chapter 9

You might guess I spent all that loooooong weekend thinking about the PLS and talking about it with my friends. But you would be wrong. I spent most of the weekend thinking about what (actually, who) I usually think about most: Forrest Charles McCann.

According to Kate, that said a lot about me and my feelings for Forrest. But I wasn't sure she meant it as a compliment.

"You fall into a mysterious office in our school, then find out you're part of a secret society. And you still want to talk about what Forrest might have meant when he said 'hey' on the bus?"

Easy for Kate to say. She's had the same boyfriend (princely Paul) since 5th grade. Not so for me. And anyway, this was a "hey" worth analyzing. On Friday afternoon, just as I was going through my PLS mail and finding out who Aretha Franklin was, the bus lurched to a stop in front of Forrest's neighborhood. He *turned around* in his seat, found me *three rows back*, said "hey," and then got off the bus. This particular "hey" from Forrest, combined with the extra effort involved in turning around, was practically an "aloha."

Unfortunately, I didn't have much of a response. He caught me so off-guard and all. I guess my eyes were focused on the front of the bus, watching him leave, so I called out "Watch your step!" That's right. Instead of saying something cool, I yelled out what it says on that big sign right next to the bus driver. I immediately ducked my head and wished I could remove it from view completely, like a turtle would.

So when I thought of the PLS and what might happen next, most roads led back to more thinking about Forrest. I could bring almost any subject back to him, so this one was no different.

Example: a toothpaste commercial with a hot guy in it. The Forrest Connection? He once told me he brushes his teeth with warm water. Weird!

Example: Someone says the football team is supposed to be really good this year. The FC? Easy! Forrest is *on* the football team.

Example: Mom says we're going to the Cedar Park shopping plaza. The FC? We will be driving *right by* Forrest's house. Hopefully, he'll be out front mowing the lawn.

Example: I've just been selected by a secret society that meets behind pink locker doors. The FC? His locker is next to mine, so maybe I could sneak him into the PLS office, just for a quick peek.

This last one is sooooo tempting because when you are in love with an 8th grade boy, you really need topics. Maybe you already know that boys, especially 8th grade boys, really don't talk that much. Oh, sure, you hear them laughing and talking with their friends or sometimes with teachers. But put one of them alone with a girl (especially a nervous one who likes him) and it gets mighty quiet. If, on top of that, you don't have any good topics to discuss, you'll hear the kind of silence that hurts your ears.

This is the kind of quiet I heard the last time Forrest and I were alone together – truly alone. We were on the 7th grade ski trip and accidentally ended up sharing the same chair lift. The pairing was a shock, but I tried to recover quickly and take advantage of our time together. As you saw with the "Watch your step" catastrophe, I can be *really* smooth around Forrest. It's hard to understand why I get so tongue-tied, really, because we've known each other for more than 10 years and our moms are friends. We've been to each other's houses and have even gone on family trips together.

Why is it that it's OK for girls and boys to be friends until 3rd grade and then everything gets totally weird? That was the year that people started saying that Forrest and I were boyfriend and girlfriend, which we were not. Not really. We were just friends who could play tabletop football or knock out on the basketball court at recess. Not wanting to answer the boyfriend-girlfriend rumors, I guess he decided to stop hanging around me and started hanging out only with the boys. Even when he came to our house, he started spending his time mostly with my older brother. And then came Taylor.

So it had been *years* since we'd really talked when the ski lift fates put us together. It was a long ride up a steep mountain on a cold, sun-splashed morning. I started slow, asking him how he was.

"OK," he said.

"I love to ski, don't you?"

"It's cool," he said.

"Your skis are really nice."

"They're rentals," he said.

"My mom wanted me to wear a helmet today, but I said no."

"You should," he said, knocking the hard plastic of the helmet on his

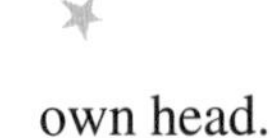

own head.

"Yeah, but I didn't want it to squish my hair because then it gets all flat and stuff."

To that, Forrest had nothing to say. What could he say, really? Helmet hair was *not* a good topic. But contrast that with inviting him to a secret office, right behind his locker wall. Now, that was a topic.

That day on the ski lift, after my hair remark, we spent the rest of the ride in quiet. I searched the landscape for something to talk about. But there was nothing to say about the tops of trees or the few clouds in the sky. We climbed higher and I could feel the temperature fall. The soft snow cushioned what little sound there was from other skiers and snowboarders below. My ears popped. Then the lift stopped, as it sometimes does when a little kid can't get on or someone drops a pole. We bobbed together on the thick cable. The quiet hung there with us and I was sure that I was blowing my one chance with Forrest. I thought about what Kate and Piper would do in the same situation.

Kate was good at telling stories and she would have reminded Forrest of something funny that happened when we were younger. There were tons of possibilities. The Halloween in kindergarten when our moms made us dress as a bride and groom. The time we had a wiener roast while camping and ate hotdogs that were charred black on the outside and icy in the center. (We called them "hotdogsicles.") I actually had plenty of material, plenty of *topics*. There were field trips and mean teachers and everything else we had seen together over the years. But not a single one of them came to mind on that ski lift.

As for Piper, well, you know what she would have done in my place. She would have told him that she liked him, flat out. And then she would have looked at him through the curls of her long eyelashes. He would have melted, as most guys do. But me, I couldn't even glance in his direction, let alone attempt that chin-down, gaze-up thing Piper does. I refocused my energies on what I'd say when we hopped off the lift at the top. I sooooooo wanted to say something like "Have a great run" or "See you at the bottom." But I ended up saying nothing. Why? Because at the top of the hill, someone took my breath away. She was waiting for Forrest, her fur-trimmed hood the perfect frame for her heart-shaped face. It was Taylor Mayweather.

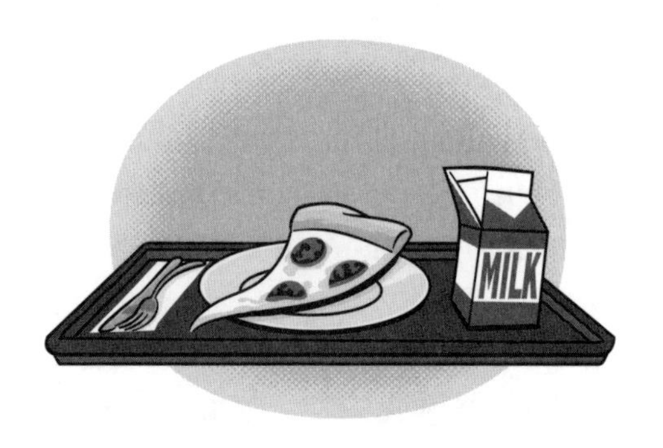

Chapter 10

Our plan for Monday was this: We would have our own pre-meeting, without Bet, at lunch. This gave us time to collect our thoughts before our meeting at 1:35. The girls had given me tips and even had me practice the pink locker combination that morning. Of course, it didn't open, but just doing it right gave me confidence. It helped that I could sing today's locker combination. Thank you, Miss Aretha.

At lunch, I sat down with my pizza and milk and was ready to talk about the PLS. But it turned out that the subjects I wanted to talk about weren't the same ones on Piper's list or Kate's. (OK, I was the only one who actually had a list.)

Here's what I wanted to go over:

- None of us has an assigned room for study hall. Discuss the potential negatives.
- What happens if we're in the secret office during a fire drill?
- Ask the group: Can I show someone (like, say, Forrest McCann) the PLS office as long as I don't give out the combination or discuss our work as prohibited in Rule 4?

But Kate and Piper wanted to get right to work on M.G.'s question.

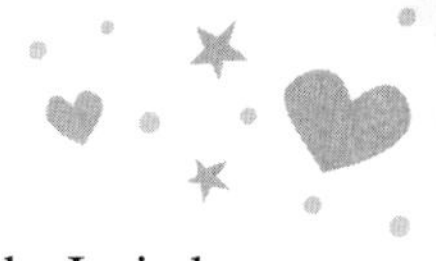

Great, I thought. No-period girl has to give advice about periods. I tried to stay very quiet and took tiny bites of my pizza so I could be chewing every time there was a break in the conversation.

"I got mine in 6th, so I think we should tell her to start worrying if she doesn't get hers by the end of the year," Piper said, spearing a forkful of her Caesar salad.

"I don't know. I don't think we should be telling her to worry," Kate said. "We should just tell her to hang in there. You can't schedule it like a dentist appointment. Periods happen when they happen."

Kate looked at me knowingly.

"Yeah, but shouldn't she go to the doctor if it, like, never comes? Maybe there's something wrong with her," Piper said.

They went back and forth for a while and couldn't decide what to say to M.G. When they turned to me, I either pointed to my chewing mouth or kind of shrugged. But as the conversation went on, I started to feel a little better. The truth was, here were two girls who had their periods, and they didn't know what to tell M.G. So me not knowing was beginning to seem like less of a big deal. Of course, this was also a problem because if we couldn't give M.G. a good answer, maybe we would get kicked out of the Pink Locker Society.

When the girls turned to me for like the 44th time, I had just swallowed the last square inch of my pizza. Kate's eyes widened as they turned to me, knowing how I didn't want to talk about this one. But luckily, the rules were there to bail me out.

"Well, rule number 2 says: 'Give high-quality advice. Don't guess. Learn and share your knowledge.' We better do some research at the library or something."

"Where did it say that?" Piper asked.

"Handbook, page 4."

I held my breath, but they both agreed.

"Ugh, the library," Piper said.

"I love the library," Kate said. "We can go tonight."

"Me, too," I said. "What's wrong with the library, Pipes?"

"I just don't get that Huey Dewey System," Piper said.

"It's the Dewey Decimal System," Kate told her. "Jem and I will help you."

We stood up and, as I did, I took note of where Forrest was in the cafeteria – sitting with the other football players and Taylor, as usual. I would have to pass right by them on my way to take back my tray. I allowed myself a quick glance – long enough to notice that Taylor was not only sitting at his table. She was sharing his actual chair!

As if she knew I was watching, Taylor threw back her head and laughed like someone had said something wet-your-pants funny. I tried to look away, but just couldn't. Then, for a flash, Forrest saw me. He didn't smile, but he didn't *not* smile either. His in-between expression was even harder to figure out than the "hey" from the bus. Watch your step, I thought. Yeah, right. You know who should watch her step? Me.

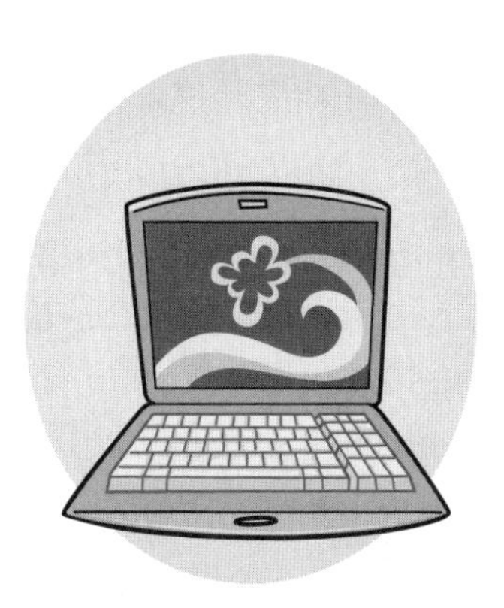

Chapter II

I sometimes psych myself up for something so much and analyze it so much, that I completely fail when it comes time to do whatever it is I'm obsessing about. Like in a monumental, crash and burn, fall out of the sky kind of way. But thank God, not today.

At study hall time, I confidently opened my real locker, waited until everyone else had drifted away, and then thrust in my hand so I could open the pink locker. I was prepared for the lighting issues this time with my key chain that has a little green light on the end. With one hand, I sent a bolt of green light toward the combination dial. With my other hand, I spelled out R-E-S-P-E-C-T. Chunka-chunka. I was in. I even closed the door quietly and stepped *ever so carefully* down the too-tall step and placed both feet securely on the thick carpet.

In fact, I was the first girl in the office and was able to look around without any distractions for about 30 seconds. What I saw made me feel once again like I was dreaming. The old-lady furnishings and the dusty tarps were gone. It was spotlessly clean and completely renovated. It looked like a ritzy hotel suite. The place could have been on TV or in the movies, like if someone was running a modeling agency or perfume

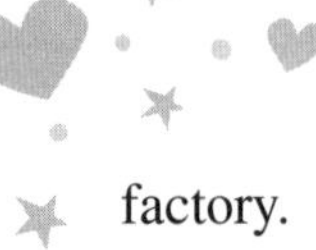

factory.

Again, I could hear music. It wasn't Aretha. It was Carole King (a mom fave). Her voice was smooth and strong as she sang about being a true friend, the come-running-whenever-you-need-me kind.

On one side of the room, there was now a U-shaped pink couch with a glass table in the center. Floral arrangements had been added to the now dust-free conference table. The old pink phone had been replaced by a sleek black model. Silver appliances gleamed from the kitchen. Lifting my head toward the loft (aided this time by my glasses), I could see a row of computers giving off their watery green glow.

The only trace of the old office was a pile of machines at the foot of the stairs. Turns out they weren't sewing machines after all. They were typewriters: super old black ones with no power cords and newer (but still old) electric ones that were aqua and must have weighed 50 pounds each.

Kate was next to arrive and she just stood in one spot, trying to take in all the changes. Piper's door opened next, but the renovations had the opposite effect on her. Piper couldn't stand still or stop exclaiming, "No way!" as she inspected each aspect of this major improvement. She found the bathroom particularly impressive.

"No way!" she said to the sparkling new faucets, stone countertops, and monogrammed hand towels. Not PLS, as you might expect, but P, J, K, and B – one for each of us.

"Who is paying for this?" Piper wanted to know. "Have you ever seen a real renovation project? It takes months. And they did this over the weekend?"

I drifted over to the conference table, where today's snacks could be found. It was oatmeal cookies (still warm) and milk (icy cold). I grabbed a cookie and looked around for the elevator. Remember the key? But even with the modernization, I still didn't see it.

Long after the golden minute passed, Bet was still not there. We went to her locker and opened it from the office side. It was dark.

"Should we, like, look for her or something?" Piper asked.

"Did anyone see her today?" Kate asked.

I hadn't, but I also hadn't really looked. The truth is I would have liked it better if it was just the three of us. Having a fourth person, who was a complete stranger, made everything more confusing. Like, at lunch today, we decided to go to the library and now we'd have to bring her up to speed and invite her along, etc.

Before we could go searching for Bet, the conference table phone rang. I picked it up and clicked the red button so everyone could hear. It was a new voice coming in crystal clear over the new phone. This one had kind of a Minnesota accent. I know my Minnesotan accents because my dad comes from MinnesoDa, where people actually do sound a lot like the characters on that old timey radio show that's on Saturday afternoons. For instance, "Ya know, if ya don't wear your ski mask today, you'll be dead before ya get to the main road."

"Hiya, girls. Things are lookin' pretty good there, eh?"

We murmured our agreement.

"Okey doke. Is everybody ready to do a little high-tech work today?" the woman on the phone asked.

"Uh, sure?" I said, a little wary.

"Ah, that's great! Why don't ya move upstairs where the computers are and put me on the phone up there?"

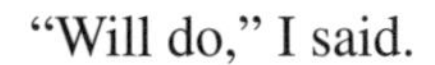

"Will do," I said.

Up in the loft, we turned on the speakerphone, and there she was again.

"Pretty nice setup, wouldn't ya say?" she asked from the speakerbox. "Ya got the Infinitrix 3000 system up here, the same computers they use in the White House."

It was awfully nice in the loft. The computer desks were whitewashed wood and the chairs were all those fancy supercomfortable ones that they sell in the back of magazines for $800. "Whose behind is worth $800?" my mother would say when she saw those ads. But you just felt important sitting down in a chair like that. The PLS computers started up quickly – nothing like the chugging old computer we had in our basement family room.

After we all sat down and logged in, the woman on the phone told us that she was going to give us a "lickety split" lesson in how to run the Pink Locker Society website. All we needed to do was learn a few basics and we'd be able to do it on our own. In other words, we soon could post MG's answer. If we had an answer for her, that is.

But before our computer lesson could get going, the woman on the phone stopped and asked us where Bet was.

"I don't see her signed in here," she said.

"She didn't show," Piper said. "We opened her pink locker, but she wasn't there."

There was silence on the other end of the line. When the woman returned to the line, she sounded a little angry.

"These meetings aren't optional," she said. "I presume someone shut her locker door after ya opened it."

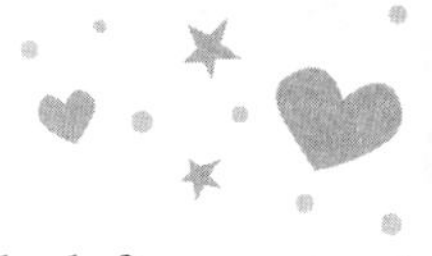

Before Piper or I could react, Kate leapt down the stairs of the loft. Slam! Kate returned to her desk in time to get a tour of the Pink Locker Society website. It had way cool music and one of those fancy intros. Then the bright pink page opened up, but it said only "Coming soon! Very soon!" Nothing like a little pressure.

The woman on the phone seemed to calm down and told us it would be "just great" if we could get our first answer up there by "Wednesday or thereabouts." That was two days away.

"Ya don't want to leave folks in the lurch, ya know," she said.

Piper mouthed "We are dead."

Kate waved her off and asked her another question about what it meant for something to be "live" on the website. She explained that "live" meant something had been published on the website. It was there for everyone to see. No one would be able to benefit from our advice if we don't get something live, she said.

It wasn't impossibly hard – as I feared – to run a website. Or at least it didn't seem so when this woman was explaining it. The site – www.PinkLockerSociety.com – was already designed for us. It was like a set of blank pages that we needed to fill. We created test questions and answers and watched them instantly fill the front page of PinkLockerSociety.com.

Kate asked: Q. How much wood can a woodchuck chuck?

And I answered: A. As much as Forrest McCann tells him to.

And *voila!* It was on the front page of the PLS website. We quickly deleted it so no one would think we'd lost our minds.

You might think Piper, no fan of the library, would have hated computer training. But don't let her fool you. She's scary smart, especially with technical stuff. She also typed way faster than any of us and was on her best behavior.

But just as the woman on the phone was finishing our training session and showing us how to log off, Piper went off topic.

"Can I ask you something?"

"Sure ya can, hon," the voice said.

"Who are you?" Piper asked.

"Oh, my, well, ya probably guessed by now that I'm a former Pinky myself. Graduated in '71. Now I run my own computer company out here in Silica Valley. Got awful lucky, I did, when the Internet took off," she said. "You guys were probably in diapers when I started my company."

"Isn't it Sili-*con* Valley?" Piper asked, which was kind of funny because it's usually Piper making these little mistakes with words. My mother calls them malapropisms, but I don't throw that word around because I didn't want to sound like a geekball.

"Sure, sure. What you said."

Piper gave me her "what the…" look, but pressed on.

"Can't you say who you are or which company you own?" Piper said. "Or why the PLS was shut down?" It seemed like a rude question, I thought. Maybe they did something wrong?

"That happened after I graduated. You can call me…Jo," she said, and then switched topics, telling us how to shut down our computers. She also directed our attention to the conference table downstairs where we'd find a pink laptop we could share and take with us to the outside world.

"Just don't lose it and don't let anyone else see it," she said. "Now, let's start a website!"

With that, Jo was gone, too. By now, we knew enough to check our mailboxes on the way out. Good thing we checked. A bunch of new questions had come in since Friday. I guess I shouldn't have been surprised, but two of them were similar questions about periods, including one from another 8th grader. So I wasn't the only one! Weird body changes, boys, problems with friends, too much homework – these subjects came up a lot. There was even one in there about a girl with really big boobs! She wrote:

This is going to sound weird, but my boobs are ruining my life. They are ENOR-MOOSE boobs. Biggest in the whole school.

I stood only a moment in the dark of my locker, eager to get back into the light and read the rest of her question. Now, how could **that** be a problem? I wondered. I should have stopped longer to listen for people in the hall. If I had, I might not have walked right into Taylor and Clementine's big fight.

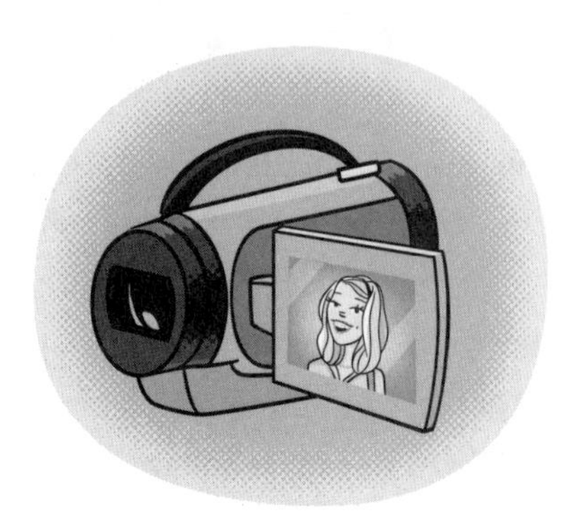

Chapter 12

Taylor's ever-present sidekick, Tia, was holding the big TV light and working the video camera, as she always did for the MSTV broadcasts. Taylor was this year's anchor for Margaret Simon TV, our in-school channel that was beamed into all the classrooms once a week, whether you liked it or not. Last year, Clem was the anchor and, it seemed, she was not ready to give up her spot. She had mostly used the privilege to film "Clem's Crib," a reality show starring…guess who.

"There's no rule against someone being anchor two years in a row," Clem told Taylor, getting right in her face. "We should have an *experienced* reporter, not just someone who does stories about kittens."

"Those kittens were found – and rescued – by me. That's a story!" Taylor shot back.

"And on top of it, I was way out of town when you guys had your supposed meeting," Clem said.

"Not my problem," Taylor said, flipping open a gold compact to check her lip gloss.

MSTV was organized as a student club and loosely overseen by our art teacher, Ms. Russo. She also does the school plays, teaches

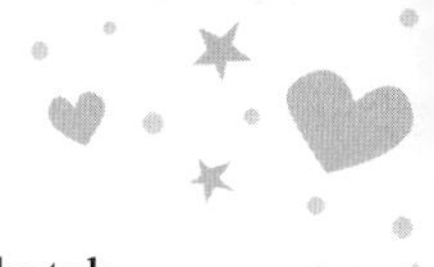

interpretive dance, and once brought in a live sheep for us to sketch. She's a free-wheeling sort and lets the kids run the TV show, literally.

Clem being Clem probably expected to get the anchor job again, no questions asked. No one looks better on camera, that's true. But the gossip around school was that Taylor grabbed control at a summertime meeting for kids interested in the TV club. Clem was in Bali on a photo shoot, apparently. With Tia on Taylor's side (Tia knows how to work the camera), what else did she need?

When I popped out of my locker, I'd like to say Taylor and Clem were so locked in battle that neither one noticed me. No such luck. Clem did look rattled, though. Her face – usually a porcelain pale – looked pink and angry. But it was Taylor who saw me first, lowering her compact to get a better look. When my two feet hit the floor, I looked up, and she looked right into my baby browns. Tia's video camera light illuminated Taylor so that, from where I was, her white-blonde hair glowed like she was an angel. Tia cut the light and Clem spun around to see me, too.

"What were you doing in your locker?" Taylor asked, a dimwitty smile spreading across her face.

"I was just … getting stuff," I stammered.

"With the door closed?" Taylor asked.

"I'm late," I said, breaking into one of those fake trot-runs. I acted like I had somewhere to be, but the first bell hadn't even rung yet.

"There's your next big story, Taylor," Clem said, "people who hide in their lockers. Film at 11." Then Clem tossed her stick-straight hair and left Taylor and Tia alone in the hall with the video camera running.

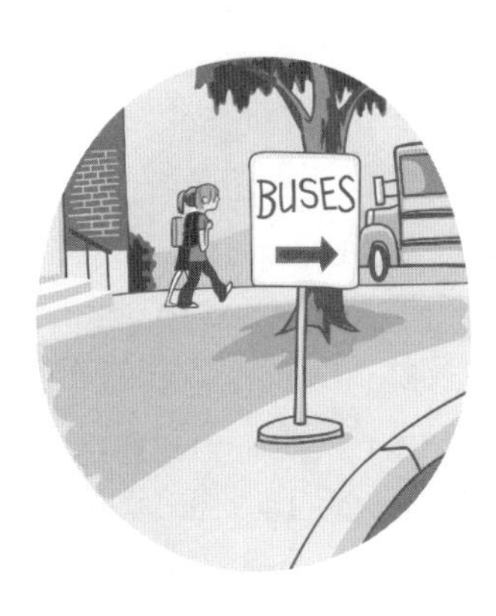

Chapter 13

Bet was waiting for us outside at the end of the day, while the buses stacked up against the curb. I knew she was short, but she looked even smaller next to the buses. Her black hair was swept back in a red headband. She wore black pants with skinny legs, and a red denim jacket. Around her ankle, I could see a tiny gold anklet with a red stone, probably a real ruby, that dipped down over her delicate anklebone. Her face looked brittle, like it might crack, and she held her head as if there were a book balanced on top of it.

"How was the meeting? Please, excuse me for not being there. Sincere apologies."

"Where were you?" Piper asked, a little too pointedly.

"I…I had something I needed to do."

"You missed computer training," Kate said.

"Oh. Well. I'm not sure I will be very good at this, anyway. Maybe I could just do office tasks. Stuff envelopes or answer the phone?"

"The phone might ring once a day and no one stuffs anything," Piper said. "Well, Jemma stuffs her bra, but I don't think she needs help."

Piper hugged me around the shoulders to show she was kidding.

"You're hysterical," I said in a monotone, then I turned to Bet.

"Maybe you don't want to be part of the PLS," I said, watching for her reaction as my words hit the air.

Bet's brown eyes looked into mine. She looked hurt. You would have thought someone had just accused *her* of bra stuffing.

"Jem, don't push her out the door," Kate said.

Kate seemed fine about not including Bet in our lunch meeting, but now good-deed Kate was in the house.

"I'm not pushing her out the door," I said. "I'm just saying the whole thing's optional."

Knowing I already hurt Bet's feelings, I continued, trying to soften my position.

"I mean, it is a lot of work, and it *will* leave less time for studying."

This time, Bet kept her eyes squarely on a crack in the sidewalk at her feet. The truth was, I would have liked to push her out the door, the pink locker door. But Kate, being Kate, insisted.

"Bet, we're meeting at the college library at 6:30 to do some research. Meet us there and we'll fill you in."

As I walked to my own bus, my worries quickly switched from Bet to something else. What if Taylor had already whispered into Forrest's ear about me? "Psst. Jemma is so weird. She hides inside her locker!"

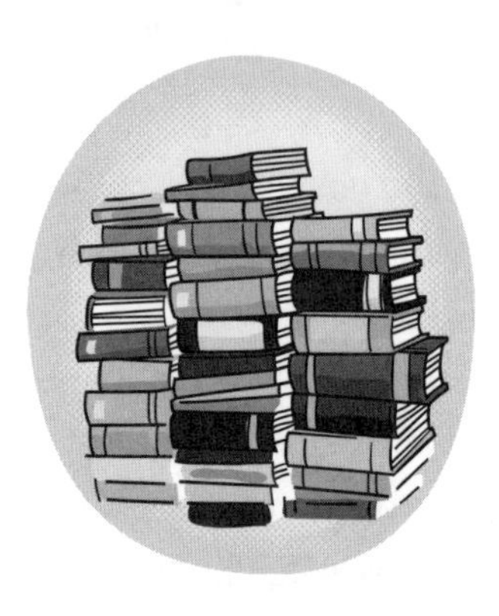

Chapter 14

Bet didn't show at the library, and I could tell Kate blamed me. Kate almost always does the right thing. If you have a friend like Kate, you know how it is. I love her for being honest and true and kind. But I sometimes don't like how dishonest, untrue, and unkind I look compared with her.

Could I have been more welcoming to Bet? Sure. I probably should have mentioned that I'd actually been to Thailand with my parents. That's what a friendly person would have done. It's what Kate would have done if she had recently been to Bet's homeland. It's probably what any normal person who wasn't me would have done.

Kate being Kate knew this, but she didn't bring it up. What should I have said? "Hey, great country you have there – the food rocked"?

I did love Thailand, but I couldn't bring myself to make this connection with Bet. It felt like giving something away. If I told her I was there, I'd end up telling her my dad's an environmental scientist who travels all over. It was more than I wanted her to know.

At the library, it looked for a minute like Piper wouldn't come either, but she finally arrived and we picked a study carrel away from the other students working so quietly. Kate's dad is a history professor, so not only can we look at books and study among the college girls and guys, but we also can check out actual books. This perk helped my real aim when visiting the college library: to convince everyone there that I was a college student. My Hello Kitty backpack didn't help my case, but I stowed it under my chair and tried to act mature.

We searched the library – and online – for information about periods. It turns out that, on paper at least, periods are pretty complicated. In books, people call them a hundred different things: menstruation, menarche, menses. (I've heard it called "Aunt Flo" and "the curse," which it definitely is not because I'd be so glad to finally get this particular curse.) And the book explanations for what actually went on inside were often technical ("the shedding of the endometrium" blah, blah, blah) and did not help us answer M.G.'s question at all. But finally, after searching a bunch of books and websites, we had some information for her – and me.

Piper, Kate, and I were feeling good now that we had an answer for our first client. I couldn't tell if I was just relieved over the comforting information we'd found about periods or if I was happy to be able to help someone. It was nice to think of M.G. out there feeling better after she read our answer.

"This could be actual fun, I think," I whispered across the table.

"Yes, but what do we tell the girl with the enor-MOOSE boobs?" Kate whispered back.

"That's easy. I know all about that," Piper said, pushing her chest in our direction. Then, in dramatic fashion, she shared her three tips for girls blessed with big bazooms:

1. Do the cleavage check. Stand in front of a mirror and bend over. If you can see down your shirt, don't wear it.
2. Wear a supportive bra that's the right size.
3. If someone looks too long at your chest, say, "Yo, my eyes are up here."

After that, our giggle-snorts made one thing very clear: We were not college students. Piper laughed out loud and then Kate tried to muffle her laugh in the crook of her arm. Unfortunately, the sound came out anyway and was amplified into a kind of farting noise.

Then Kate said "What if you really could see out of your boobs?" If that were true, Piper said, then some boobs might need to wear glasses. That was about all I could take. My laughter turned into hysterics and I slid down in my chair – trying to be funny at first – but then I fell to the floor. People started turning around in their chairs and I expected a librarian to come over and shush us. But there was no shushing librarian because this is college, after all.

OK, so after that performance, no college guys were going to ask for our phone numbers. But we did now have two answers ready for the Pink Locker website. We still had a little time before my mom picked us up, so Kate headed over to the archives and told Piper and me to take up the third client question about whether to tell your crush you like him.

We couldn't find a single book in the library that gave advice about the tell-or-not-tell issue. But Piper and I agreed that people have been asking this question for a long time. Even really old stories, like the ones my mom sometimes reads to me out loud, seemed to be about love – both hidden and revealed. Piper reminded me that this plot had been well-explored by several TV shows. In the past or present, I was not at all sure whether it was better to love someone secretly or to reveal that love and possibly – oh, quite possibly – get your heart squished.

I also wasn't sure that Piper would be much help on the subject. Sure, she knew what it was like to be a crush, since so many boys liked her. But I didn't think she had a Forrest McCann rolling around in her brain all the time. It was as if she read my mind with what she said next.

"You know, everyone has a Forrest McCann," Piper said.

For a minute, I worried that she said she also liked Forrest, which would pretty much eliminate me from contention in this lifetime. But then she continued.

"I like someone right now and I don't know whether to tell him," Piper said. "On the one hand, you want to know if he likes you, too. But what if he doesn't?"

Whoa. We shared more common ground than I thought. Who was her Forrest McCann? I ticked off the cutest boys in school but none was the one. And what about Jamie Welch, who was supposedly her boyfriend right now? Finally, she gave up the name.

"It's Jonah Zafron," Piper said.

"You're thinking of telling *the movie star* Jonah Zafron that you have a crush on him?"

"Don't you think he would want to know?" she said, doing that chin-down, eyelashes-up thing she did so well.

Before I could remind her how old Jonah was or that he already had a girlfriend, Kate returned from the archives with a stack of papers. She slapped it down in front of us and together we read the headline of the Pink Paper, published in October 1976. In big, blaring type, it said: PINK LOCKER SOCIETY IN DANGER! But the headline was all we could read. Every line of the article had been blacked out.

Chapter 15

If you were to visit www.PinkLockerSociety.com, here's what you'd see today. Ta-dah! Our first answers for our first clients:

To M.G., the girl who was worried about not getting her period:

Dear M.G.,

You can breathe a sigh of relief – plenty of girls do NOT have their periods by 6th grade. The first period happens during puberty, which can start between age 8 and 13. But the key word is START. Some girls are starting at 8 and some are starting at 13. After it gets going, puberty takes a while and runs over a few years. Most girls get their periods between the ages of 10 and 15. Everyone is different, but it usually happens about two years after your breasts start developing.

Unfortunately, periods don't come by appointment. You won't know until it arrives. If your first period (aka "Aunt Flo") arrives for the first time when you're at school, don't panic. Instead, be prepared by keeping some supplies (a couple pads) in your backpack or locker. If you need help, ask a friend or a female teacher. If you stain your clothes (this hardly ever happens because first periods are usually light), wrap a sweater or sweatshirt around your waist until you can change.

And we understand how you feel about your period. It's OK to want it and it's OK to not want it, even at the same time! Anything new is weird for a while. It's also more than OK to talk to your mom or another girl/woman you are close to. If you need some questions answered, why not ask someone who knows Aunt Flo quite well! Think pink!

The PLS

I keep track of all my major successes in life. The list is not that long, but I'm happy to say that I think today is one of them. We answered not only M.G.'s period question, but also the one about big boobs and the one about crushes. You already know Piper's advice about getting your chest stared at. Thank you, Piper! After a lot of thought – and a conversation with Kate's older sister – we offered this advice to the girl who wrote that she kinda-sorta wanted to tell her crush about her true feelings.

Dear D.M.,

Crushes are called crushes for a reason. They can hit you hard! People have been asking your question for hundreds of years and the answer is not crystal clear. It can feel wonderful to learn that your crush likes you, too. Imagine Christmas morning and your birthday combined. Woo-hoo! But when the person doesn't have a crush on you, it can feel like a dozen rainy Mondays all at once.

The good news is that crushes are like playing make-believe. It's probably been a long time since you did that! But crushes are a way of imagining, thinking about, and even testing out what it's like to fall in love. So it's up to you if you want to take a risk and see if your crush likes you, too. Are you feeling brave? Or maybe you'll decide that your crush is more fun kept as a secret. The only thing we know for sure is that this won't be your last crush. Think pink and happy crushing!

The PLS

We felt really good to get those answers up there. But we felt even better when we went to the PLS office, signed on to our computers, and saw that the website got more than 100 visitors by lunchtime! I even heard some girls talking about it in the bathroom. Not only that, but lots of people sent us email *thanking* us. Here are a few:

OMG, you guys soooooo rock. I was very worried about "Aunt Flo" and now I know exactly what to do when she makes her first visit. Thank you! Thank you!

Signed,

A not-so-nervous anymore 7th grader

I have had a crush on someone for a long time and now I feel mucho bettero.

Your friend – BBallGRL96

Thank you, PLS! I am feeling less worried and much more unshy now about periods. I think I might ask my mom about it. After all, she was young once. I've seen pictures!

Keep up the good work,

M.G.

D.M., the crush girl, and the girl with the big boobs hadn't written back yet, but I hoped they liked our answers. Walking around school, I felt different. I couldn't put my finger on it, but I figured it was at least a first cousin to being popular. What I felt like was a celebrity, even though no one knew who I was.

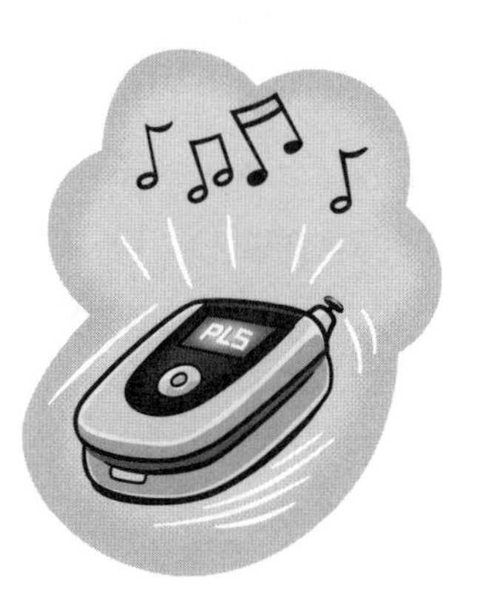

Chapter 16

A person can get used to almost anything, my mother often says. She's even written a poem about it – one of the many I don't completely understand. On one hand, it's great that people can adapt and get used to new stuff. Kate, Piper, and I quickly got used to the fact that we were part of a secret society. In the same way I trundle off to the caf for lunch at 11:47, I now go to my locker every day at 1:35 and crawl inside. (And try not to get caught on the way out.)

Beforehand, I write that day's pink locker combination in the palm of my left hand. No one ever asks why I've inked myself with words like "BLOOM," "LEADER," and "TRUTH."

In our headquarters, I grab the daily snack (the fudgy no-bake cookies are my favorite) and we take care of business. As predicted, PBBs account for most of our inquiries. But there have been other questions on the fringes. One girl asked about what to do if you're afraid to get your ears pierced. And we've even had a couple questions from boys. They mostly want to know about girls and what to do if you like someone – eerily similar to the kind of questions girls ask!

We're getting so much "business" now that we're working during every study hall and tapping away on the pink laptop during evenings and weekends. (Great, but not so great for my grades!) Somehow word has spread and our "customers" are writing from places far beyond Margaret Simon Middle. Some apologize that their English is not so good and the ones from Great Britain are funny. They say "holiday" instead of vacation and call cute boys "fit" instead of "hot" like we do here. We're getting so many questions now that Piper rigged our laptop to call our phones with a special ringtone when we have a new one. At first, it was fun hearing the first few bars of "Respect" (duh-nuh-nuh-duh-nuh-*nyah!*) every time a new one came in. Now, it's a little scary because it's a sign of how much work is piling up.

Demanding as it is, I squeezed the PLS into my life. The PLS work gets done just like volleyball practice (now that I've gotten "used to" running those endless laps around the gym). And also like volleyball, being in the Pink Locker Society makes me feel good, as if I'm an important part of something. I love it when I hear people buzzing about the website or wondering who runs the Pink Locker Society. I've even seen "The Pink Locker Society Rocks!" written on the inside of one of the girls' bathroom stalls. And I took out a book from the library recently and found a Pink Locker Society bookmark inside. It was like an ad and said: *They're cool and confidential. Ask and the Pink Locker Society will answer!*

That's me – I'm cool and confidential. It's like a very excellent secret and even though I've had trouble keeping secrets before, I've gotten used to keeping this one. But this secret would be more fun to keep if it were just between me, Piper, and Kate.

Kate, of course, has been Kate through this whole thing. She has done her best to include Bet in the PLS, even though – if you ask me – Bet is a half-time, half-hearted member. She misses a lot of meetings and hasn't answered a single question from any of our readers. She barely says anything, just nods a lot and hangs close to Kate.

She doesn't really talk to me since that day by the buses. I guess Bet has gotten used to being the new girl, on the outside of everything, used to being so quiet you hardly know she's there. Even though I see her almost every day, I guess I have gotten used to one more thing: not being Bet's friend.

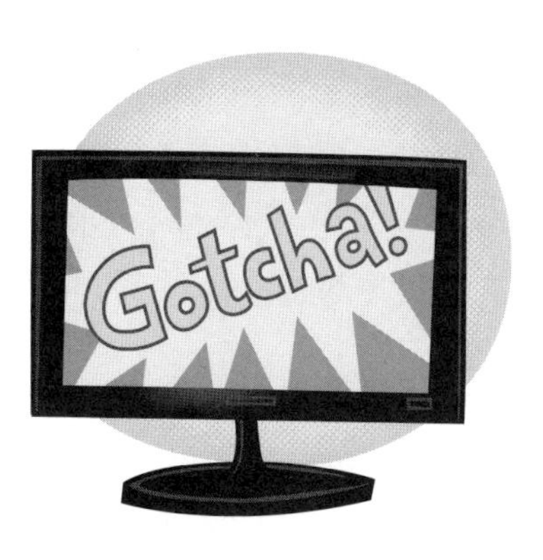

Chapter 17

Fridays have always been my favorite days and I know I'm not alone. It's the last day of the school week and all that. But Fridays are not my favorite anymore. On Friday, in last period, everyone must turn attention to the TV because we are forced to watch Margaret Simon TV. Last year was one thing, watching Clem parade around during "Clem's Crib." "Here's my shoe closet, here's my at-home foot spa for pedicures…" It was sometimes dull, but not an unacceptable way to waste 10 minutes.

Now that Taylor's the anchor, everything has changed. Of course, since she's Forrest's current girlfriend, I didn't exactly long to watch her cutie-pie face. And coincidentally, Forrest called my name on the way into class today, but by the time I turned around in my seat, Mr. Ford said, "Face front, let's be courteous during Taylor's broadcast." When I looked back again at Forrest, he just laid his head on his folded arms, like he was going to take a nap.

Probably spurred on by Clem's criticism, Taylor had dramatically changed her approach to her broadcast. Gone were the kittens. Music boomed loudly in the intro to a new show she called "Gotcha!" It began with a scene from a recent football game, the cheerleaders all posed in a perfect pyramid. Perfect at least until Marina Testarosa wobbled from her perch at the very top and they all came tumbling down. The class laughed a little and the camera turned again to Taylor who smiled in a pink turtleneck and said “Gotcha!”

From there the report went to a video of Clem Caritas standing in front of the girls’ bathroom mirror, putting on lipstick and trying different smiles – the first one big and movie-star-like and the next one shy and closed-lipped. Then she winked at herself. “Gotcha!” purred Taylor again, this time pointing a jaunty finger at the camera.

And so it went on for 10 uncomfortable minutes, watching people caught on secret video. Even though he said nothing, I could tell Mr. Ford was getting annoyed by the way he sighed and shifted in his squeaky desk chair.

“It’s funny, right? I think it’s really funny,” Taylor explained, live to the class.

That seemed to give them more permission to laugh and they did so with increasingly volume with each new clip. The one of Mr. Updike, the janitor, chasing a groundhog around the front lawn drew a real hoot. Hardly anyone laughed though when the camera zoomed into the cafeteria, zeroing in on a long lunch table where Bet sat alone, eating delicately from her lunchbox.

“Gotcha!” Taylor said, rubbing her eyes and putting on a fake sad pout.

Just as I was gathering some sympathy for Bet and hating Taylor just that much more, I saw a familiar row of lockers emerge on the screen. The sound was muted, but I could see Taylor looking angrily at someone, who turned out to be Clem. It was their big fight about who should be anchor.

Then, the camera moved in close to catch me slipping out of my locker and stepping a foot gingerly on the linoleum tiles. My face can't hide my surprise and, with cheeks flushed pink, I hustle by the camera until Tia could do nothing else but record my fast departure down the hall.

Back to Taylor, who this time said, "Gotcha! Locker Girl!" and narrowed her eyes into a "Could she be any weirder?" kind of look.

My mom often says that we don't absorb difficult things all at once, but rather in stages. My first stage here was breathless shock. I would have gotten up to leave the room, but I was paralyzed in place. Everyone looked at me, some of them still laughing. Forrest made no eye contact.

The second stage was an incredible desire to act – to do something. Running away wasn't my first choice, once I had a moment to think. What I wanted to do most was lift Taylor – desk and all – and fling her like a whirlybird out the classroom's third-floor window.

The third stage was trying to make sense of it all. Of course (my brain finally reasoned) Tia had the camera rolling that day in the hallway when I caught Taylor and Clem fighting. And what it captured was not just the catfight between them, but my odd re-entry into the hallway. I was now the weirdest girl in school, worse than Bet eating alone or Clem smiling at herself in the bathroom. I was someone who spent time inside her locker with the door closed.

Thankfully, Taylor's segment soon ended and Mr. Ford grumbled something about moving along because the buses were already lining up. I started to gather myself but I felt like I was moving in slow motion, having to think about each step I took. Pick up backpack, step with the right foot, now with the left. Kate and Piper ran up to me after class, but I couldn't even talk.

"What a beast, she is – like that Jerry Springsteen on TV," Piper said.

"It's Jerry Springer. Springsteen is the singer," Kate corrected, "Are you OK?"

"No," I said in a weak voice. I walked with great effort to my bus, like I was walking through deep, deep snow.

To my surprise, someone was standing at the bus's door, waiting for me. It was Forrest.

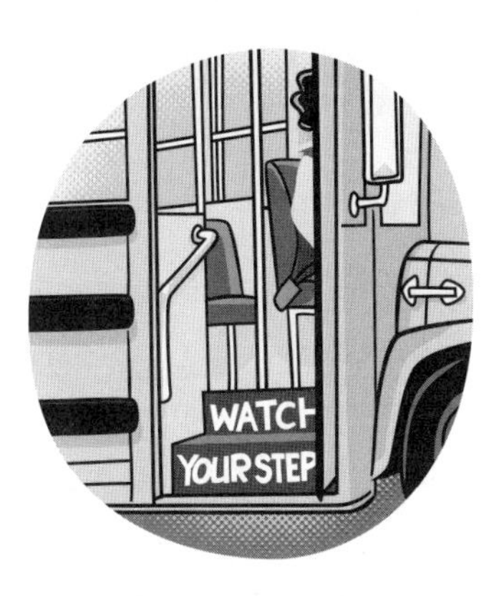

Chapter 18

If I told you that Forrest not only waited for me, but that he *sat with me* on the bus, would you believe it? How is it that the very worst thing and the very best thing happened to me within the same 20-minute stretch of time?

"I was trying to tell you before class," Forrest said from the window seat.

Taylor had shown him the video, he told me, and he knew how embarrassed I would be, how embarrassed everyone in it would be.

"She's trying to prove she deserves to be the anchor this year," he said, as if making excuses for her.

"Well, whatever it takes, I guess."

"I know. It's mean. I told her it was mean, but she said that's journalism."

I tried to talk more, but I was afraid I might cry – cry because I was so embarrassed and cry because I was sitting so close to Forrest and I wanted him to stay there forever. I stared ahead at the green vinyl seat and bit my lip. He was quiet for a long while and then he said, "Can I ask you something?"

I turned to him and watched a lock of beachy brown hair fall over his eyebrow. If I touched it, what would he do? Slap my hand? Let me? "Yes, you can ask me something," I said.

"Why were you in your locker?"

It was a fair question. Of course, I knew I shouldn't tell him. At this point, my bent knee was either touching his knee or the electricity between us was just making it feel that way. I told him I couldn't tell him, but someday soon I could *show* him.

Now it was Forrest who gave me one of those quizzical looks. It was a little like the one Taylor shot at me from her "Gotcha!" tape, but it was ever so much kinder. Not to overanalyze it, but I hoped that look said, "We're friends, maybe even friends with potential."

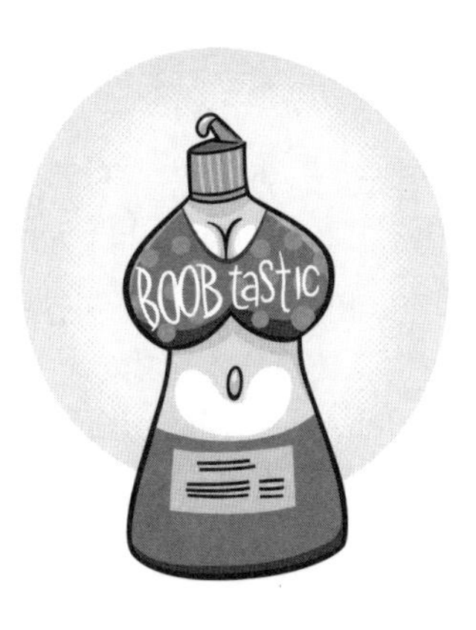

Chapter 19

All weekend, I confess, I thought of Forrest and his sweetness to me and hoped that it was something more than just him being a good guy. I wanted to know if he had tried to warn anyone else about "Gotcha!" If it was me and only me, then that surely meant something. I also weighed – and reweighed – the idea of sneaking him into the Pink Locker Society offices. I said I would *show* him, didn't I?

My membership in the PLS may well be the coolest thing about me, so I really wanted him to know. And what an adventure it would be. We'd have a shared secret to tie us together always.

Once inside I could show him how the website worked, offer him a snack from the fridge, and tell him how the society mysteriously ceased to exist in the 1970s. Wasn't that a mystery to unravel? I saw us chatting together on the couch and then maybe I would ask him about Taylor and why he was with such a miserable girl. Then, maybe he would ask my advice and I would say, "Why don't you go out with someone who really cares about you?" And then he would figure out that that someone was me.

Of course, there were problems with my plan. I wasn't supposed to let other people into the office. I could be kicked out of the PLS, which – even though only a handful of people would ever know – would be worse than getting caught climbing out of my locker. Then there was the issue of me finding the courage to actually say that Forrest should be going out with someone else, ahem, me. With Forrest, mostly I stuttered and stammered and backed myself into dumb conversations. Remember the ski lift?

But whether I would have the courage or not, maybe I should be more like Kate and stay on my best behavior. The rules were not to take anyone into the PLS.

I was tossing and turning all this in my head on the way into school on Monday when Kate and Piper stopped me dead in my tracks. They pulled me into the back of the empty auditorium. Look at this, they said, and opened the pink laptop to reveal the Pink Locker Society website. Only now there was a huge ad on the page for *Boobtastic – the amazing miracle product that makes mountains out of molehills!* The ad popped up, nearly swallowed the whole screen, and it put up a fight when you tried to close it.

The Boobtastic ad was particularly bad news because that very day we had answered a question from a girl who said she was uneven in the boob department. "Lopsided" didn't know what to do about it. Our advice had been good and reasonable, but it was now pretty much drowned out by Boobtastic.

"Is it – some kind of cream or pill?" I asked.

I was curious in more ways than one.

"It doesn't really say," Piper said, sticking out her chest, "but I'd be afraid to try it."

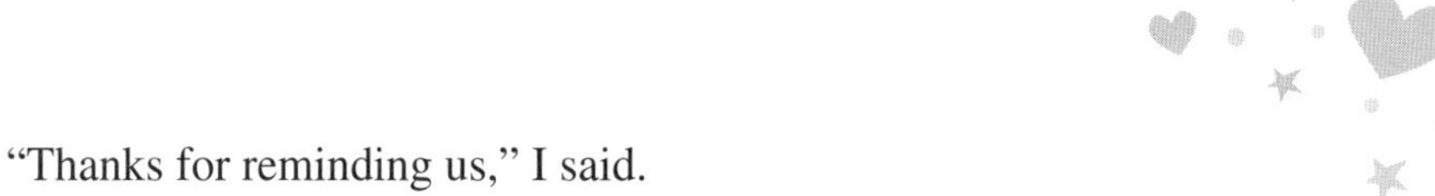

"Thanks for reminding us," I said.

"Whatever it is, it's cash payments only – $19.95 plus shipping and handling," Kate said. "I can't believe everybody will see this."

It did seem to give the wrong message. By now – after researching the answer for our uneven friend – we knew that being a little lopsided wasn't anything to be alarmed about. Girls grow at their own pace – in my case, horribly slowly – and sometimes unevenly. We looked into it and found that, usually, your lefty and righty even out or the difference is so small that no one notices.

But this ad made our answer look like a joke, as if this weird product were the answer, almost like we were making fun of the people who wrote to us. It didn't stop at Boobtastic. Our answer on freckles was paired with an ad for *Freckle Free, the fantastic, life-changing product that can erase freckles!*

Even the girl who wrote in to say she was in love with her older brother's best friend was not spared. We gave her our best advice on crushes and suggested she get to know him as a friend. But the ad that popped up urged her to buy *Love Potion Plus, the fabulous, fast-acting product that makes any boy fall for you!* Now if that were true, I'd buy a gallon of it and spray it, like a fog, over Forrest.

"Who did this?" I almost yelled.

"It doesn't matter who, we just have to fix it," Kate said.

Piper suggested we use the PLS-SOS. I was impressed. She had read the handbook, which said in case of emergency we could text to an emergency phone number. She whipped out her red phone and texted only this: What R these ads?!

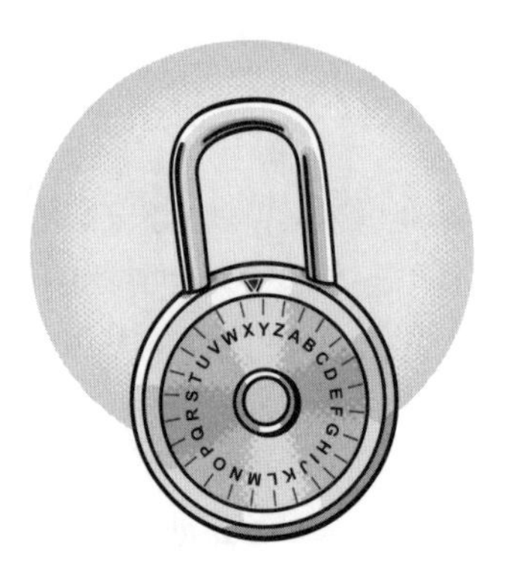

Chapter 20

At 1:35, a little breathless, Kate and I rushed into the PLS offices. We overlooked our snacks and ran upstairs to answer the ringing phone. Piper and Bet were already there.

It was Jo on the speakerphone.

"Hiya, girls, what's the emergency?"

"It's the ads," Piper said. "We were surprised to see them?"

"Oh, them. Just a few. Ads are everywhere on the Internet, right? You've seen ads before."

"True," Kate said, "but these seem weird. What in the world is Boobtastic?"

"I'm not sure. I think it has some botanicals in it – freesia, maybe?" Jo said.

"It's not just Boobtastic," I interrupted. "It's all this stuff that goes along with the questions we're answering – Freckle Free, Love Potion Plus. Do they work?"

"Caveat emptor," Jo said.

"Caviar what?" Piper said.

"Caveat emptor is Latin and it means 'Let the buyer beware.' People buy what they want and take risks on stuff all the time."

I had to admit it was true. My mother was always making fun of those ads for wrinkle-reducing cream and wondering who believed a $100 tub of goo would make you look younger.

"Maybe the products somehow work?" Piper said.

"Exactly!" Jo said. "Customers want options."

I had never thought of the girls who read our site as customers. She went on to say that we had more customers than ever – about 10,000 visitors over the last week. That was way more than the 100 visitors we had when we started.

But Kate was not buying the stuff about options.

"Why are we bothering to research and write good answers and then tell them to buy some dumb cream?"

No response from the phone. Then Bet spoke up, quietly.

"Did you ever buy something off the TV? I, myself, have been disappointed."

There was quiet on the other end of the phone. Finally, Jo cleared her throat and said, "Do you think that those fancy offices you have were free? And what about the ongoing expenses, computer maintenance, that pink laptop you're carrying around?"

Her voice sounded weird, more gruff, like maybe she just developed a bad cold. But this "money doesn't grow on trees" speech was familiar to all of us. We'd heard it from our parents. I didn't want to lose anything, like our computers, the monogrammed towels, or even the snacks. From there, our questioning kind of fizzled and Jo reminded us that we had work to do.

"A dozen new questions came in just in the last hour. Chop-chop!"

she said.

We knew. Just then our phones started emitting that familiar ringtone: duh, nuh, nuh, duh, nuh, *nyah!*

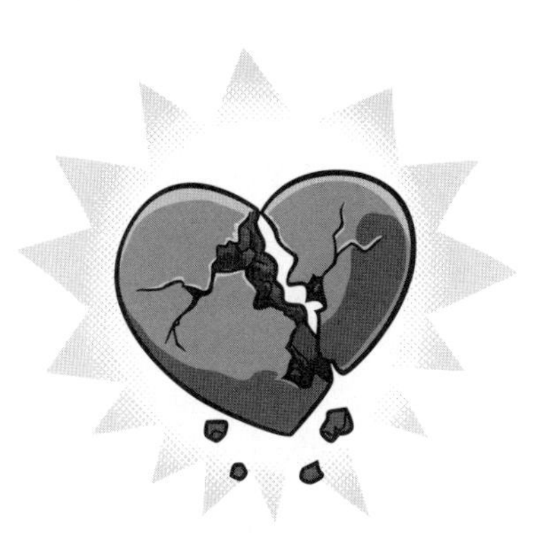

Chapter 21

Did you ever hear the expression "Be careful what you wish for"? I wished the PLS would be a smashing success and it was. But now our success was starting to work against us. We received more and more questions each week, even with the ads, and it was tough to answer them – and answer them right – and still keep up with schoolwork. I, for one, had a huge English paper that I hadn't even started. Bet was always saying she missed meetings because of school. (It showed because she was the only one who seemed to be keeping up her grades.) Even Piper and Kate – who always did well – were feeling the strain. We all had to turn our phones off or be constantly bothered with new alerts that we had more questions sitting in our Pink Locker Society emailbox.

So we decided to split the responsibilities of the PLS. Instead of all of us going to the headquarters every day at study hall, we would each take turns going alone one day a week. But on Fridays, we'd all go. It made sense and meant that I could actually study during study hall three out of five days a week. We still didn't have assigned rooms for study hall, so we tucked ourselves deep in the reference section of the library. No one suspected a thing.

It was sometimes a little creepy going into the PLS office alone, but mostly it was quiet and I got more done when there was no one to distract me.

So far, I had answered questions about bad breath, stinky feet, and accidentally tooting in class. Embarrassing stuff was becoming my specialty. After the "Gotcha!" incident, I guess I was the school expert. Actually, I couldn't have answered these questions from the Gross Department without our school nurse, Mrs. Wolff. Somehow it wasn't embarrassing to ask an embarrassing question when it wasn't about you. It was easy for me to ask questions about periods, for instance, since mine was still nowhere to be found. There was no end to what girls wanted to know: Could you swim with your period? Do periods hurt? Should I eat certain foods during my period? I got answers for every one.

"Gotcha!" didn't appear again on MSTV after that first week. Principal Finklestein pulled the plug, but unfortunately, only temporarily. Taylor told anyone who would listen that he wanted to kill it permanently, but Ms. Russo convinced him that anything created by a student for MSTV was free expression, *protected by our nation's Constitution*, and he didn't want to get into a First Amendment battle, did he? For such a laid-back teacher, Ms. Russo got fired up about being able to say what you want and create what you want. Not to knock the Constitution, but this made me pretty mad because why should Taylor be able to express herself by embarrassing me and everyone else on her video?

I'm happy to say Principal F. agreed with me and they forged a compromise. They would open the competition for the MSTV anchor spot to *everyone*. All a person had to do was submit a video and it would be judged by a panel of people including Ms. Russo, Principal F., and a couple actual journalists from the local TV station and daily newspaper. We students would get to see each person's video and would have "input" into the final choice, but Principal F. also talked a lot about "appropriateness." Ordinarily, I would have been up in arms. It's our TV station, shouldn't we get to be the final judges? But in this case – knowing Principal F. was no fan of "Gotcha!" – I was fine with it.

I even thought for a moment about submitting my own video. I would have loved to interview everyone who was embarrassed in Taylor's first episode. But then I thought it would just draw more attention to stuff that everybody, including me, would have preferred to forget. Not that I had any time for another extracurricular activity. I was overbooked and overwhelmed with volleyball, homework, and all my Pink Locker website responsibilities.

Some days we were so busy answering PLS questions that we forgot to eat our snack and had to grab it on the way out. For a while there, I stopped noticing what music was playing. The last time I went in alone, I made an effort to listen. I sort of recognized the song, but the girl – was it a girl? – was nearly screaming. I checked the CD (they were still putting them in our mailboxes once a week) and it was someone called Janis Joplin. She was singing about someone not only breaking, but *taking* pieces of her heart. I could sort of understand.

I mean, on the one hand Forrest was all "I wanted to warn you" about the "Gotcha!" stuff. But on the other hand, he was still with Taylor – even still sharing a chair with her in the caf. And it was just like Janis sang it. My heart felt like it was disappearing one tiny little piece at a time.

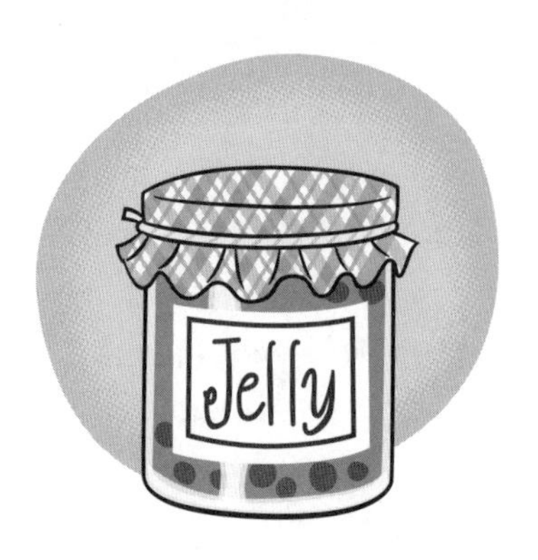

Chapter 22

Let me start by saying I know it wasn't right. But the more I prepared, the more it seemed like it was OK. I actually wrote myself a script for what I would say. Memorizing my lines made me feel sort of confident. Of course, I had to guess at what Forrest might say back. But I figured I knew him pretty well. I mean, did anyone else know that his favorite jelly was the mixed fruit flavor – the kind you usually find only in those packets at diners? But knowing his jelly preferences was not enough to get me through the 21 minutes we spent alone in the PLS offices.

I planned it out like a crime. Splitting up the Pink Locker work created my window of opportunity. On Wednesdays, I went to the office alone. I hoped there would be a good snack and that something soft and romantic would play over the speakers. Was it possible, I wondered, to make a request?

But when the time came, my head was too filled with love, fog, and electricity to listen for the music. I hoped that day's pink locker combination would be "LOVE" or at least "FLIRT." It was "CONFIDENCE." Forrest was easy enough to capture. He was at his locker, right next to mine, just before study hall started. He often spent his study halls in the gym working out. No one would miss him. When the hall crowds thinned, I leaned over to Forrest and spoke my first scripted line, "I can show you now."

Lesson No. 1 to all you girls out there who really like a boy: Don't count on him remembering everything you ever said to him. You may think you have inside jokes and your own secret code, but you probably don't. Forrest just looked startled and said, "What?" And when I said it again – "I can show you now" – he said "What?" again. Maybe I should have started with something like "Hi."

Anyway, this led to me doing a lot of overexplaining, burbling on about that day on the bus and "Gotcha!" and how I said I would *show* him someday and now I was ready to *show* him. Finally, he seemed to recognize me and there was a glimmer of something on his face that went back to that day on the bus. Seeing that he was already semiconfused, it was not the best time to show him the pink locker in my locker, swing open that pink door, jump in, and pull him in with me. But that's what I did.

I remembered to reach back out and close my real locker door, just as I noted in my script, but that was the last time I followed my prepared lines. It wasn't that Forrest said something so different from what I had guessed he would say. It was that Forrest said nothing. Standing together inside the PLS offices, he looked a little afraid. I think he was mad at me. Later, I had to feel sorry for him. On my first trip into the PLS headquarters, at least I had a little warning and time to get mentally prepared. Forrest just got pulled in, kidnapped almost. His face started to soften after I explained where we were and what this was all about.

"I'm the Pink Locker Society. I mean, I'm *in* the Pink Locker Society.

This is our office. You know what the PLS is, right?"

Now Forrest gave me a look of disbelief, but then I pulled him toward the loft to show him the computers. And then I whipsawed back to the table to get a snack – cheese and crackers today.

"Want some?"

"No," Forrest said, his first word.

"Well, maybe if I had mixed fruit jelly for the crackers?"

OK. Have you heard me loud and clear? Assume no inside jokes or secret code. He looked at me as if I were wearing my underwear as a hat. Zero recognition. Maybe he had moved on to something more exotic in the jelly department.

I continued to talk too fast and move too fast, but Forrest seemed to wake up when I turned on the computer up in the loft and he saw me working on the website.

"I've seen this," he said. "Taylor goes there all the time."

Great. He's said 10 words to me and one of them was "Taylor."

"What is it supposed to be about?" he asked.

You can imagine that my answer was a little awkward. I like Forrest *a lot* so I don't exactly want to discuss PBBs with him. I mean, for me, he's the second "B" after all. What I did tell him was that girls need to know a lot of stuff as they get older and the PLS helps them get answers to embarrassing questions.

"Mmmmm," he said.

Should I count that as word 18?

"Like about growing up, changes, and crushes and stuff," I said.

After that, his words came out in a string that was too long to count. He had some questions:

"Who's in charge of this?"

"How did you get picked?"

"Where is that music coming from?"

Until then I hadn't noticed, there was music. It was more stuff my mother liked. Joan Baez was singing "The Night They Drove Old Dixie Down."

"Why is this a girls-only thing? Don't you think guys have questions and need help, too?"

"What's up with the ads?"

And finally, the toughest one: *"Why did you bring me in here?"*

Because I was so overexcited, I didn't know where to begin. Finally, Forrest and I had such a very fine topic before us. It was spread out like a feast and I didn't know what to try first. I had so much to say. But before I could choose, something in the room changed.

Joan, who had been into the "Nah-nah-nah-nah-nah-nah" part of the song, suddenly stopped. In all of my hours in the PLS offices, that had never happened. The music always played. Forrest looked at me oddly and then something worse happened. We heard a sound like a closet door sliding open and shut. Then I heard low talking – and it sounded like it was coming from behind the wall.

I could feel my breaths coming faster and I wanted to run. But I held my hand up, motioning for Forrest to stay still and let me listen. I could make out just this much before the fear took hold: A gruff-sounding man said, "I told you to pick the little foreigner and now she's the only one following orders. It's time to take care of this. Enough pussyfooting around here."

It was then that I bolted for the door and Forrest followed right behind me. I shut the pink door and we were wedged together in my locker. Even as my heart was pounding with fear, I stopped a moment to savor the smell of Forrest's hooded sweatshirt. I inhaled slow and deep and then Forrest said, "Open the door. I'm suffocating." I let out my breath and lifted the latch.

We stepped out of my locker and I hoped there would be time to analyze and consider what had just gone on. Was I about to get thrown out of the PLS? Is Bet some kind of double agent for these guys? Could we perhaps go somewhere so I could answer Forrest's questions in detail? For instance, maybe the PLS should start answering boys' questions, too. It would have been a good time to pull out my script. But Forrest quickly gathered his stuff from his own locker and said he had to get going. And then I could only watch him hustle down the hall, cleats in one hand, toward the gym.

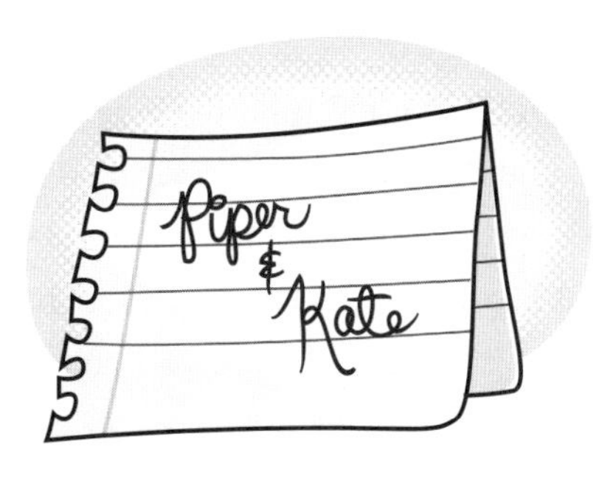

Chapter 23

Some stuff that happens sticks to you forever. Here's what I mean: Piper will always be known for losing a shoe on the bus in 7th grade and having to walk around at school with one red sandal and one bare foot. A boy who liked her held the sandal out the window to be funny, but the bus scraped against a tree branch and it slipped out of his hand. Of course, he felt terrible and told the bus driver to go back but he wouldn't. So Piper hobbled through school for several class periods, at least until her mom got there with a new pair of shoes. Her barefootiness lasted only a few hours, but she acquired a nickname (Barbie Barefoot) and the story blanketed the school so that, by lunch, everyone knew.

But that sticky story benefits Piper. The whole reason it happened was because Jake Blume (a cute boy) was trying to get her attention. Second, the "Barbie" part of the nickname suggests that Piper herself is cute in a Barbie-perfect kind of way. But my sticky story – getting caught in my locker – was not such a win-win.

Being inside of your closed locker does not suggest that cute boys like you or that you're pretty. It's just weird. Until today, I had pretty much shaken my "Gotcha!" moment. Sure, there were people who would always remember it, but I had not acquired a nickname and after the initial whoop-dee-doo, it kind of passed.

Fast forward to today, three weeks later, when I opened the Pink Locker website. What I saw made my stomach feel like I had just taken a long ride down a roller coaster hill. It was "Gotcha!" right there on PinkLockerSociety.com. Someone had added a video player to the PLS site and with just a click of your mouse, you could see the original "Gotcha!" show starring me and my locker. For some extra fun, you could get a sneak peek at the next round of embarrassing clips that Taylor was getting ready for the MSTV anchorperson contest.

How did "Gotcha!" get added to our website?

I immediately texted Kate, even though texting in school is against the rules. Her message back: "Yikes."

My anger about this swelled like one of those waves that carry surfers for miles. I'm talking a Hawaii-big wave, not one of those two-footers at the Jersey Shore. Mainly, I was mad about the "Gotcha!" thing. Now, people all over the country – maybe even the world! – would get a chance to laugh at me. I'd be a celebrity, but just for being a doofus. I mean, what the pink?

But there was more. I wrote it all down on a sheet of loose-leaf paper when I should have been doing proofs in Mr. Ford's geometry class. In my note to Kate and Piper, I listed all the stuff that went wrong with the Pink Locker Society since we started.

Remember how excited we were at first? Then came so many questions we couldn't handle them all, stupid ads for stupid products, and now mean videos of people doing dumb stuff, particularly me!

I continued with three itemized points:

1. When we told Jo how we had too much work to do, she made us feel guilty and said, "Well, who do you want to let down this week – the girl who's afraid to get her ears pierced or the one who doesn't know how to tell her mom she needs a bra?"

2. When we complained about the ads, she said they were paying for our offices and even our cookies and milk! And when a few kids wrote in to say the stuff didn't work, Jo said only that "individual results may vary." (Big surprise – Freckle Free doesn't fade freckles and Boobtastic does not grow bigger boobs.)

3. And now, they have added those "Gotcha!" tapes for all the world to see. Why? Why? Why? And what do "Gotcha!" tapes have to do with upholding the grand and noble tradition of the Pink Locker Society? What happened to "be a friend to all" like the handbook says?!!!!!!!

I probably shouldn't have been so energetic about those last exclamation points. The pencil tapped loudly against the hard plastic of the desktop: Slash dot! Slash dot! Slash dot! As I finished that last dot, Mr. Ford leaned down and said, "What are you working on, Jemma?"

Oof. Great. I'm writing about being embarrassed and I embarrass myself again because Mr. Ford calls me out for writing notes in class. Worst of all, he took the note.

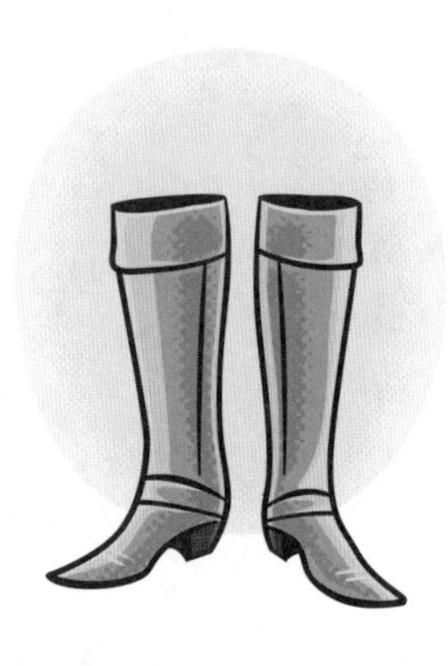

Chapter 24

Without my note, I had to just tell Kate, Piper, and Bet all of my complaints about the Pink Locker Society. Turns out, they were getting pretty fed up, too. At lunch (yes, Bet was eating with us now), Bet said she felt "sick in my stomach" thinking about how kids might be buying Get Taller Now vitamins and toothpaste that promised to make kids' teeth straight without braces.

"What if some people in my country bought these potions? Twenty dollars is a lot of money there," Bet said.

"It's a lot of money here if you only get $10 a week for allowance and you just bought $50 boots," Piper said.

This made all of us look at Piper because she seemed so genuinely angry, and she was wearing some really cool emerald green boots. Kate, of course, was having her own problems with the whole thing. She said she turned to her mom for advice.

This made all of us turn to look at Kate because no one had told their mom about the Pink Locker Society. Remember the rules? Tell no one. But then Kate reminded us about the whole legacy thing. Turns out, a legacy means something that gets passed down and Kate was a "legacy

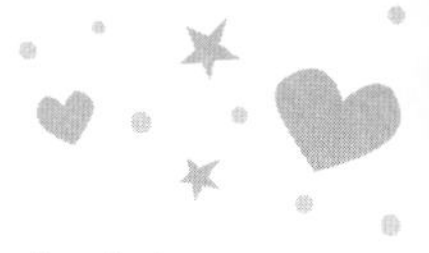

member" of the PLS. We sat there looking dumb until she made it plain.

"My mom was in the Pink Locker Society."

Mrs. Parker?

We exploded with questions for Kate.

What was it like back then?

What did they do when there was no website?

Why were we picked?

Does she know Jo or that grandma lady who called us the first day?

Are we doing a good job?

Did she always keep it a secret?

Why did the Pink Locker Society shut down?

And who decided it should reopen?

Can she help us get this junk off of the website?

Kate tried to answer them all. Her mother told her it had been a great honor and she loved serving as a "Pink Locker Lady." According to Mrs. Parker, girls have always wanted to know pretty much the same stuff, Kate said. But back in the day, the questions were submitted through a secret box in the girls' locker room in the gymnasium. They typed up answers and printed it on something called a mimeograph machine. Then they distributed the Pink Paper around the school. They left them in the girls' bathroom and in certain other hiding places.

Kate was a great source of history, but she couldn't answer any of our questions about the Pink Locker Society today. And her info on the history had its limits.

"My mom doesn't know why they decided to start it up again," Kate said. "And she doesn't know Jo. She said she must have come before or after her."

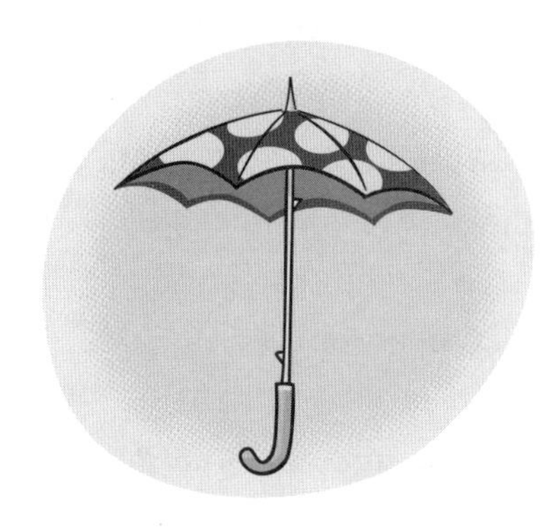

Chapter 25

For a minute there, I lost my head. Of course, it involved Forrest and it involved me thinking too much. Before we could ask Jo some questions about "Gotcha!" I started piecing together bits of information. I put them together in a completely wrong way, I guess. I got to thinking that it was quite a coinky-dink that I just showed Forrest the PLS offices and the very next week, his girlfriend's stupid "Gotcha!" videos end up on the website. Remember he said she was on the site all the time? So maybe Forrest told her everything and she somehow horned her way into the Pink Locker Society. Thanks a lot, Forrest!

My biggest mistake was confronting him with all this before I had completely thought it through. Nor did I calculate just how goofy people start acting if they are low on sleep. (I had been up late the night before trying to finish my English paper.) Just as I was about to go into the PLS offices at study hall, I started accusing him at his locker. I said a lot of "How dare yous" and "How could yous" and I waved my arms for dramatic effect.

He tried to get some words in, but I kept interrupting. I've never before seen that look on his face. It was kind of like he looked when I

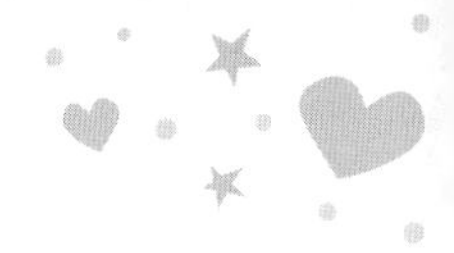

pulled him into my pink locker, but 25 times worse. He looked angry and confused and kind of embarrassed to be part of such a scene. When I finally ran out of steam, he spoke firmly and slowly. They sounded like the last words he would ever say to me.

Jemma.

I.

Don't.

Know.

What.

You.

Are.

Talking.

About.

****

I'm sure no one will be surprised to learn that the next day, a cold, autumn rain poured down over Margaret Simon Middle School. What a perfect match to my mood. It rained all the while I waited at the bus stop – the kind of rain that gets you even under your umbrella. And there's no keeping your feet dry. Cold, wet toes were just one more complaint I could add to my All That's Gone Wrong List, with my attack on Forrest ranking as No. 1.

Jo finally answered our PLS SOS, though it was clear she had had enough of our questions. Of course, Forrest had nothing to do with the addition of the "Gotcha!" clips. Jo said that Taylor herself had emailed them to the site. (Funny, I never saw this email, but whatever.) Jo said she put them on the website because it makes people want to visit it more often.

"Any traffic is good traffic," she said.

I pointed out that I was actually in one of the clips and that I was caught exiting my locker, something that might be a clue about where the PLS secret offices are. There was a long silence from Jo, who then said, "Just keep your mouth shut and it will be fine."

"Any more questions from anybody else?" she asked.

We said a lot in the glances we traded with each other, but spoke not a word. After Jo hung up, we silently went to work on that day's questions. But it was hard to concentrate on other people's problems (a girl who feels too tall, another who is worried about her grandma's breast cancer, and a third whose best friend just stole her boyfriend). Piper passed us a note that said, "I have an idea."

When we were safely back in the school hallway, she told us more about it. In her spare time, Piper had been playing around with some software that blocks pop-up ads. If kids knew how to get this same software, it would block the bogus ads on the PLS site – or any site, she said.

"We've got to do it before someone else gets ripped off," she said.

Her plan was to answer a very unusual question – one no one had actually asked us: How can I block annoying ads on my computer? Our answer would guide kids to this solution and *voila!* the ads would go bye-bye. While she was at it, Piper said she was programming the pink laptop so we'd get *all* the email that came into the Pink Locker Society, instead of just the ones Jo wanted us to see. That would explain why I never saw the one from Taylor "Gotcha!" Mayweather. And probably why we never saw a single complaint about the so-called miracle products.

Piper's idea was clever, for sure, but I was a little scared. What would Jo do once she found out? Maybe she wouldn't notice? No, she'd notice. I wondered if we'd get kicked out of the PLS. And then, sadly, I wondered if that might be the best thing for us anyway.

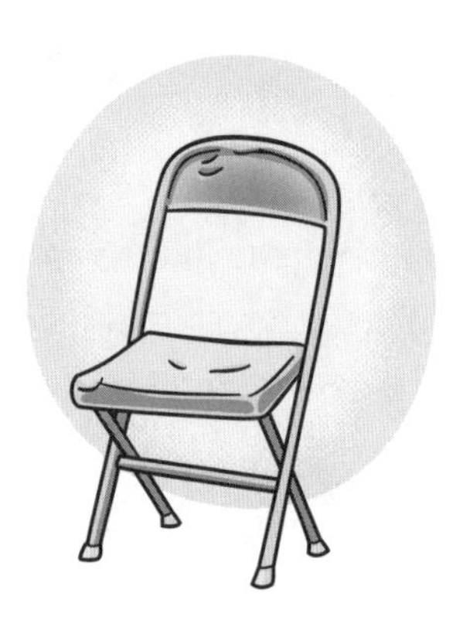

Chapter 26

At first, it seemed like we had gotten away with it. We published Piper's easy-to-follow ad-blocking directions with a big batch of questions. There were so many! Girls wanting more information about tampons, others who wanted to know about shaving their armpits, and one girl who asked how old you needed to be to dye your hair. We heard nothing from Jo for more than a day, enough time that we exhaled and started congratulating ourselves on solving this problem for so many of our loyal fans.

We all started to feel better about the website. On Friday, we piled into the PLS offices with a renewed good attitude. That day's pink locker combination was "BOLD." I was still dreading the MSTV anchor contest scheduled for that afternoon, but even that couldn't break my stride. Maybe Taylor would lose. And I prayed she would not show that locker clip of me again.

"Whoa, what's up with the lights?" I heard Kate say from across the office. The lights in the PLS office weren't off completely, but they were very dim. We finally found each other at the room's center. There was something coming from the speakers, but it wasn't exactly music. It was

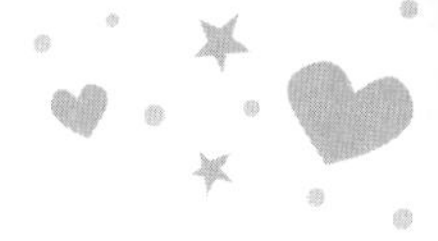

wordless, kind of like those recordings of whales talking to each other.

"Something is peculiar here," Bet said.

"Très peculiar," Piper said, reaching for whatever was on the snack tray. Was it a brownie or a scone?

"Mmmmmm, but these rock. Have one," she said, giving one to Bet. Piper and Bet had been getting cozier lately and I didn't like it much. It made me remember what that weird guy behind the wall said about only one of us "following orders." But I couldn't tell anyone about that comment because I couldn't tell anyone about that day and what I was doing in there with Forrest McCann.

Bet took a tiny bite and said she was too nervous to eat. Then they both scurried upstairs to the computer loft.

"Hey, what happened to our cool chairs?" Piper yelled down to us, leaning over the railing.

Kate and I shrugged.

"Looks like somebody replaced them with those rank folding chairs from the caf. No lumbar support there," Piper said, before spinning around and getting to work on the computer with Bet. I couldn't hear what they were saying, but they were excited and giggly.

Downstairs, Kate and I compared notes.

"Why is Bet acting so weird?" I said.

"Didn't she tell you? She's competing in the contest this afternoon to be the next MSTV anchorperson."

"Bet?"

Well, I can't say I was rooting for her, but I was rooting more for her than I was for Taylor. And no one wanted Clem Caritas to be the star of her own show again.

"Maybe they're saving money on the lights because no one is looking at the ads anymore," Kate said. "And the chairs? Did they sell them on eBay?"

"It's kind of a haunted house effect with the whales, don't you think?" I said.

"Sorta, but who's afraid of whales?"

Am I the only one who thinks whales are a little creepy? They could swallow you whole after all, but I kept that tidbit to myself.

That's when the phone rang. Bet and Piper bounded down the stairs together and announced they were "done." Done with what? Bet wanted to leave early because of the contest, she said, and Piper went with her to do her makeup. That left Kate and I behind to answer the phone. There was no hello.

"Just what do you girls think you are doing?" Jo barked into the phone.

Kate and I looked at each other so long without saying anything that she said it again.

"That stuff we're selling isn't good," Kate said softly. "It's not helping anyone."

"Ya don't know that," she said. "Ya don't know anything ya think ya know, believe me."

"Can't we just answer the questions without the ads?" I asked in a miniscule voice.

"No ads? Sure, we'll ask Santa Claus and the Easter Bunny to pay our bills."

Just then, on their end, we heard some rustling and Jo said something to someone else. It sounded like she had her hand over the phone.

"Girls, can I just remind ya to stick to your work and leave the grownup decisions to the grownups? Or before you know it, the Pink Locker Society will go out of business entirely."

She hung up and I felt like crying. When she saw me about to speak, Kate put her hand over my mouth. On a sheet of notebook paper, she wrote, "We don't know who is listening."

Together, with the whale calls still playing, we went back to work and kept at it until the bell rang.

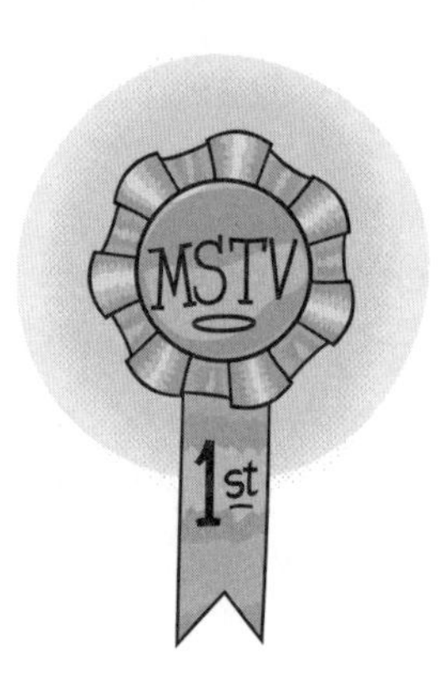

Chapter 27

Assemblies go one of two ways at Margaret Simon. They're either horribly dull so that everyone gets into a half-comatose state or everyone gets sooooooooo into it that it's completely rowdy and Principal Finklestein threatens all kinds of punishments until it's over. The anchorperson contest turned out to be one of the wild ones.

It was kind of like one of those reality TV shows. Everyone was competing and there was something at stake, even though it wasn't a million dollars. It probably helped that there was a convenient villain. The crowd, to my delight, was rooting against Taylor and the "Gotcha!" show. She appeared first with another round of clips. Thankfully, none were of me, but I can't imagine Nelson Todd and Ian Zimmerman were too pleased. They were captured sitting in the nurse's office after they disturbed a nest of yellow jackets on the baseball field. Nothing like showing the world a face full of red, swollen welts.

At first, it was really quiet as the "Gotcha!" video ran. A few people laughed at Nelson and Ian, but then Taylor's clips got a little too insider-y. They were inside jokes, I guess. While the clips showed a long sequence of sandaled feet, for instance, I could hear Taylor and

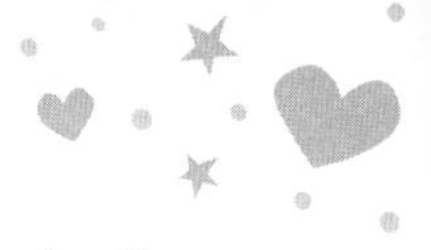

Tia laughing, but no one else was. Then came some footage of what I guessed was Taylor's dad sleeping on the couch. He was snoring, which was kind of funny, but it wasn't even particularly loud or dramatic snoring.

Just when I thought it might just be me who didn't get it, a faint sing-songy chant arose. "Bor-ing!" "Bor-ing!" "Bor-ing!" It grew louder and I joined in, after checking around to see if Forrest was near enough to see me. Principal Finklestein intervened, of course, and when Taylor's segment ended, there was some brief, polite applause. A few people booed, which made me worry a little bit about Bet. What if her show wasn't good?

Clem was next. She put a new spin on her old show, "Clem's Crib." This one was "Around the World With Clem Caritas." In it, she showed the camera her favorite fashion souvenirs – a batik sarong from Bali, a sickly expensive purse from L.A., some rose soap "someone really lovely" gave her in Paris. You get the idea. Clem received no boos, and at the end people cheered for her so that her name stretched to two syllables. "Cleh-em! Cleh-em!" But I think they cheered because she was fun to look at no matter what she was talking about.

The other entrants received pretty much the same excited response. There was the kid who did magic tricks. Not bad, actually, but it didn't seem like he knew enough tricks to do a weekly show all year long. One girl performed a one-woman play: "Me and My Dog, Sophie." It was cute and funny, and, afterward, people in the audience shouted "Woof! Woof! Woof!" I thought she might win. A dog in cute little people clothes would be a hard act to follow. Bet was next.

Her tape began to roll and I felt a shiver as I saw images of the Pink

Locker Society website. What was she doing – blowing our cover? My heart was beating so loudly I heard it in my ears – kunga, kunga, kunga. The audience was hushed. Then the point of her story came into focus.

"The Pink Locker Society is performing a vital service for girls," Bet told the camera in a serious anchorperson voice. "But what about the products it advertises? Creams that claim to improve a girl's figure, lotions that promise to erase freckles, and even potions that are supposed to make someone fall in love with you. Do they work? And where does the money go if you buy one of them?"

Whoa. I was cool with what she was doing. And amazed that she had answers. No matter which product someone bought, Bet said all the cash-only payments were sent to the same address in Hyattsville, Maryland. I never noticed that. She even went there in person and had video of the building! It wasn't a factory. It was just a rundown house and no one opened the door when she knocked.

Then came the real shocker. Bet, wearing a simple navy blue dress, told the camera that she interviewed actual girls who bought the "miracle" products. I expected to see some of the less popular girls in school, some 6th graders for sure. But when the tape cut to an interview, it was Piper, our 8th grade Piper! Sounding both sad and angry, Piper said she bought a product called Super Skin. It promised no more pimples and perfect skin in just two weeks.

"I just hate when I get a pimple. I try covering them up with makeup, but it never helps. I wanted good skin like girls in magazines have."

Personally, I had never noticed Piper had particularly bad skin. But the camera focused on a picture Piper had obviously taken of herself. She had red spots on her nose, chin, and cheeks.

"Super Skin did nothing for me. I think my pimples got worse when I started using it."

Piper ended up going to the dermatologist who gave her some stuff that did help with her acne, she said. Not a miracle cure, but an improvement. Bet then asked the doctor to analyze the tube of Super Skin and she found it was nothing more than petroleum jelly – pure grease! The doctor explained that Piper's acne probably did worsen because petroleum jelly would clog the skin's pores.

"I feel dumb and I wasted $20," Piper said. "But maybe by telling the world, I'll help other people avoid my mistake. Before you spend your money, ask the doctor for help with pimples."

The segment ended. Bet had saved the title of her proposed show for the end. She called it "On Your Side? You Bet!" The crowd erupted in what else, "You Bet! You Bet! You Bet!" They were louder cheers than before. Some people were on their feet. It didn't hurt that the show featured Piper, but it was more than that. Even I had to admit it.

Bet deserved to win. To my surprise I was plain happy for her, especially when Principal Finklestein announced the winner and she took the stage. She looked out on all of us and smiled – not a fakey anchorwoman smile, either – a real one.

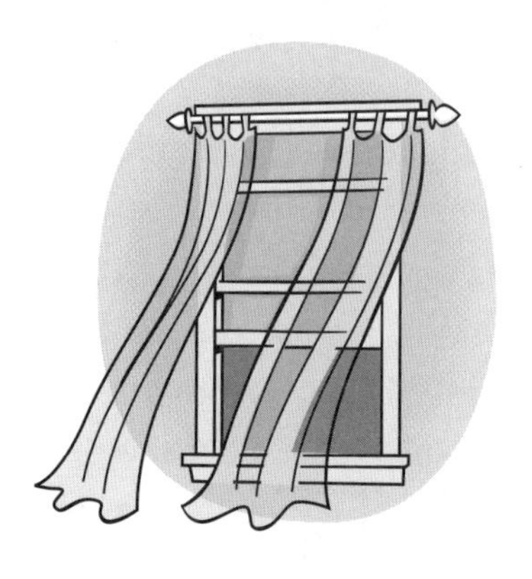

Chapter 28

It was still chilly during my walk home from school, but it was finally sunny and the leaves were changing colors in my neighborhood. I had fought my way through the crowd to congratulate Bet. I didn't go so far as to give her a hug, but our encounter was hug-like. I said, "good job" and smiled. Now, as I walked along, it made me smile to myself and I felt an extra spring in my step so that my hair swung back and forth more than usual. What I didn't know was that I was striding confidently down the sidewalk toward a kind of disaster.

When you're away from home, do you ever think about what is going on in your empty house? Maybe the cat is up on the kitchen countertop, where she knows she's not supposed to be. Or you might imagine your mother's stained glass lamp in the living room and how it changes color as the sun dips behind the roof of the house after lunch. Important calls could be coming in for you from people too shy to speak to the answering machine. Or the breeze from your open window could be slowly detaching one of your taped-up posters from the wall and silently sliding it under your bed.

I admit I think of these things, and it's always a peaceful scene at home when I'm not there. Bad stuff doesn't happen in my imaginings, just tiny adjustments, witnessed by no one. It was in that mindset that I walked home, enjoying the layers of my good mood. Not only was it cool about Bet's victory, but Piper revealed what she and Bet were working on earlier that day in the loft. They rigged the Pink Locker Society website so that anyone who visited would be sent first to Bet's website (she already had one!), where they could see her report on the bad products. Of course, I was afraid of what Jo might say, but until she caught up with us, it felt good to be doing good.

My mind wandered farther the closer I got to home. I thought about how I would burst in the door and tell my mother how my grades had finally started to rise, just in time for report cards. When I had good news, I liked to start out looking very serious and down. (My mother fell for this every time, owing to her natural tendency to imagine the worst possible scenario.) Getting her all concerned first would make it all the more fun to spring the happy news on her. But dang! This was Friday and Mom didn't get home until 4:30. The good news about my grades would have to wait, I thought, readjusting my backpack on my shoulder.

Two more blocks to go: Thoughts of Forrest always figured into any thoroughly good mood of mine and this one was no different. It's true – I hadn't spoken to him since that day I yelled at him about the "Gotcha!" videos. But I had just made a bold decision as I crossed Muir Avenue. I would gather my courage and apologize to him, in person and out loud. Of course, I was worried he wouldn't accept it. It was safer to *not* apologize and still have hope than to approach him and find out he never wanted to see me again. But I was finally exhausted from not knowing. A new script was in order! With Mom not home, that was something

I could start right in on. As I turned the corner on my block, I started playing with opening lines. Nothing too clever this time, I promised myself. Just normal English.

But all thoughts of my new script washed away when my house came fully into view. A bunch of cars clustered in our driveway and lined up along the sidewalk. You welcome such a sight when you're having a party. But when you're not, you only worry that something is terribly wrong. That some of the cars were blue with darkened windows only seemed to confirm my worst fears. I broke into a run and didn't stop until I reached my front door. On the way, I passed not just my mother's car, but the bike my father rode to his office every day. I moved too fast to catalog the other cars, except one. The green Jeep, I recognized instantly. It belonged to Forrest's mom.

Our lacquered black front door was open, so I pulled on the storm door and stepped into the living room, which was filled with people. Their murmuring conversations stopped when they saw me. They were standing around like they were at a party, but without food or drinks. My mom and dad stepped out of the crowd.

"Jem, there are some…um…officials who need to talk with you," Dad said.

I couldn't really form a question, but I looked around the room and said words: "Officials." "Need." "Me?"

Then two suited men came forward. They were good looking enough to be on TV, though one had graying hair.

"Ms. Colwin, we need to ask you about potentially fraudulent interstate commerce via the Internet."

The gray-haired agent saw my startled look and translated.

"We're with the FBI. We need to know about your involvement with the Pink Locker Society."

"Did something happen? Are all the girls OK?"

"Which girls?" the first agent said.

Again, the gray-haired agent saved me.

"You mean Piper, Kate, and Bet? They're fine. They're here."

It was true. It was like when you finally see the hidden images in a picture. My friends came into view. Their parents were with them. I was less scared, but still confused, especially when I spotted Forrest in the crowd. My teacher, Mr. Ford, was there, too. The gray-haired agent introduced himself as Lee Cheever and said there was a problem with the Pink Locker Society.

"It was a scam, pure and simple," Agent Cheever said. "What can you tell us about the grownups who were in charge?"

I went on to describe Jo and the grandmotherly sounding woman, but I didn't know their names.

"They are not who they said they were. Evidently, they met someone in prison who told them about the society – a former member. Disgruntled, I guess. And they hatched this plan to make money off of kids," Agent Cheever said.

"Prison?" I said. "Those two women were in prison?"

"Not so fast," he said. "One of them's a guy."

"I knew it!" Piper said. "Jo is a guy. It makes perfect sense. Jo isn't even a girl name."

"Actually, Jo *is* a woman. Her real name is Mandy 'Flim-Flam' Sorrenson. It's the other one who's a guy. The one who talked to you the first day," Agent Cheever said.

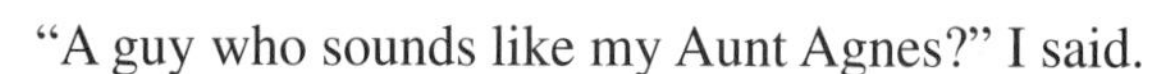

"A guy who sounds like my Aunt Agnes?" I said.

"His name is Hector Federinko. Their specialty is identity theft – stealing credit cards and the like, so it helps that he can sound so sweet over the phone," Agent Cheever told me. "But he's not your Aunt Agnes. He's big into junk products these days."

"That's what we've been saying!" I said. "Bet just did a whole thing on this today at school…."

I found Bet in the crowd, looking for assurances that I hadn't dreamt everything that happened today. I saw her and she looked deflated, nothing like she did just an hour ago.

"We know, ma'am," the younger agent interrupted. "Ms. Hirujadanpholdoi has already been debriefed."

That sounded weird until Agent Cheever said, "He means she's been interviewed."

"Ms. Colwin," he continued, "since you all spent time alone in the secret office, we just need to know if you had any additional contact with either of the two individuals. Did you ever meet them in person? Do you have any landline telephone numbers for them?"

The answer was no. He asked me question after question, but I could be of no help. I didn't know who or where these two people were. None of us had any real information, except for Bet who had tracked down that address in Hyattsville.

"This duo has made off with thousands of dollars and they could be anywhere," Agent Cheever said more to the parents than to us.

Among themselves, the grownup conversation had to do with why "in this day and age" we would have trusted people we never met before. I hated being talked about in this way. Agent Cheever also said the website

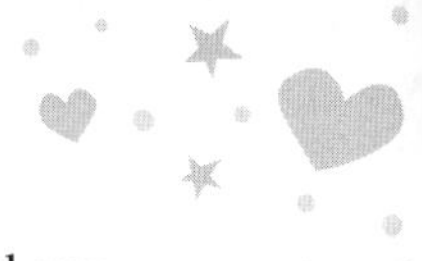

had been shut down, permanently. I looked across the room and saw Kate's eyes light up.

"We have the laptop – the pink laptop," she said.

"They issued you this equipment?" the younger agent asked.

"They, uh, gave it to us," Kate said.

"That could be very helpful. Thank you," Agent Cheever said.

Piper reached into her backpack and pulled out the computer. The young agent grabbed it and slapped a yellow evidence sticker on it. Then the agents started saying thank you to the adults and that they'd be in touch. They also said we should call if we thought of anything else.

"I blame myself," Kate's mom told the agents. "I was a part of this group 30-some years ago and I told her it was OK."

"Don't blame yourself, ma'am. These two were very smooth," Agent Cheever said. "They replicated everything about the old group. Carried on all the traditions, what with the music and the handbooks and all that."

Agent Cheever went on to say that they had managed to trick some adults, too. They talked a former Pinky into making a large donation used for the computers and the furniture. Then they sneaked in and took it all, leaving the office empty. They also convinced a teacher they were legitimate, he said. Agent Cheever did not say which teacher.

"Evidently, she was a former Pink Locker Society member herself and was responsible for the music and the snacks. Right before Sorrenson and Federinko started cleaning out the office, they locked her out, too," Agent Cheever said, but he seemed to be talking more to the adults. The grownups were, by now, looking glum and shaking their heads in disbelief.

I felt dizzy and sick. With no real destination in mind, I wove in and around the people in my living room until I was in the kitchen. Then I moved through there into the laundry room. I opened the extra fridge and thought about getting something to drink. But instead I just stared into the cool air, unable to focus on any one thing. I needed a moment to absorb what had just happened. I needed more than a moment, actually. The secret society we thought we were in was a complete scam and we were stupidly part of that scam, even if we didn't mean to be. And that is why, at 3:45 in the afternoon, my living room was filled with actual FBI agents, Mr. Ford, all my friends, the boy I am in love with, and everyone's parents.

Because I was still in this state of early absorption, I was not prepared to hear that boy call my name. But he did. Forrest was standing in the doorframe of the laundry room and looked a little like he did that day I dragged him into the PLS offices. Not scared exactly, but rattled.

"Jem, are you OK?"

I studied him for a moment like he was a ghost, probably because I often imagined what it would be like if he was where I was. Last summer, I pictured him on the seat next to mine during that long whale watching boat tour my family took. I've also imagined him at the other end of pool as I executed a perfect dive, my painted, pointed toes entering the water with hardly a splash. All that imagining made him seem not to be real, but here he was: just a boy in the doorway of my laundry room. He was standing next to the old washboard my mom hung on the wall.

I don't know how much time passed with me just staring at him. But when he repeated his question to me, I just said, "No, I don't think so."

"It's going to be OK," Forrest said. "They told my mom and me that

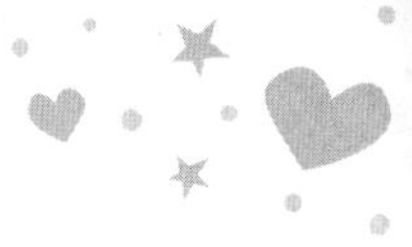

we're not going to get in any trouble. It's just that they're trying to catch those people who lied and whatever."

Then, like a bucket of cold water, it hit me. Forrest was there, being interrogated along with the rest of us, entirely because of me. I dragged him into this.

"God, they know you were in there, right?" I said. "How did they know?"

"I don't know, some kind of video surveillance that was in the school, I guess. I just told them you wanted to show me around. I told them you didn't do anything wrong."

It was then that I shivered and realized I was still holding the refrigerator door open. I turned my back on Forrest and told the water bottles and the extra milk jug that I was sorry.

"What?" Forrest said.

Then I closed the fridge, turned to him and said it – in English, in person, and out loud.

"I'm so sorry, Forrest, about everything."

Here came the pause I was so worried about. He could say anything or nothing. I held my breath because I didn't want to think about what it would be like to go to school on Monday, and all the other days that would follow, if I couldn't look forward to seeing Forrest there. But he didn't stay silent. And he didn't say he hated me. Or that he didn't want to talk to me ever again.

"It's OK," he said. "It was an adventure."

"I shouldn't have blamed you for the 'Gotcha!' thing. It wasn't your fault."

He smiled at me, the smile of old times. He smiled like that when we used to play flashlight tag and that time when we ate pizza at the Fourth of July fireworks. It was back before he was my No. 1 obsession. Years ago, he was just a boy who was my friend. Maybe that's what he still was, or could be. But before I could analyze our laundry room moment as much as I wanted to, he said we'd better get going.

Out in the living room, the grownups were wrapping up. The agents handed business cards to our parents, thanked us for our cooperation, and left. One by one, the girls left with their parents until I was left alone with mine. Usually, Mom and Dad want to talk about stuff until the cows come home. But this time, they just said, "Why don't you get ready for dinner? It's been a long day."

Never fear, the lecture came soon enough. Later that night, after we ate, my mom and dad told me that I shouldn't have been so willing to go along with strangers. Thank God, they said, that Mr. Ford turned my note in to the principal, who then called the FBI. These were bad people, what if this and what if that, my parents wanted to know. I couldn't talk, but I didn't have anything to say anyway.

After a little while, I started to cry. I think I cried some for the Pink Locker Society, which now seemed lost forever, like a dream you can only remember bits of. Though it made me seem younger than I was, it felt very good for my parents to be sitting there with me, wiping my tears away and saying what my mother always says, "This, too, shall pass."

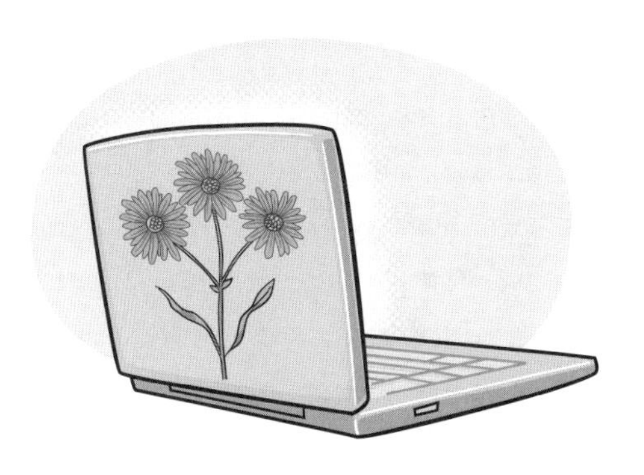

Chapter 29

It took more than a month, but I started to think less and less about the Pink Locker Society. My grades improved. Piper, Kate, and I were still best friends. We all supported Bet's new MSTV show. I started running and seemed to be good at it. Taylor and Forrest continued to be a couple, for reasons I don't understand. My mother, quoting Forrest's mom, gave me the only clue I have about the situation. Turns out, that night the FBI came over, the two of them actually talked about it.

"Vera thinks it's a bit soon for Forrest to have a girlfriend," Mom told me. "But she says something about Taylor just fascinates him."

What else do you need to know? No, I still hadn't gotten my period. But I wasn't completely a Flatty McFlat Chest anymore. And, no, I didn't use Boobtastic to make it happen.

The strips of yellow crime tape over our pink locker doors were our only reminders that we had once passed in and out of there on a daily basis. Wait, that's not true. Sometimes I would run across a 6th grade girl who looked particularly confused and think that she needed the Pink Locker Society. I didn't even have to hear her speak to know that she needed some guidance, probably because not so long ago I was that girl.

You know the one? She pushes with all her might on the door that says "PULL" in letters as big as her head.

But who would answer her now? Our laptop was gone. The website was gone and all that was left was a federal investigation. It had been weeks since our cell phones alerted us to a new question with that familiar tune: duh, nuh, nuh, duh, nuh, *nyah!*

For a while, I wondered if I was in any danger as a witness in the Pink Locker Society case, but the FBI agents said Flim-Flam Mandy was probably happy to be anywhere we – and the FBI – were not. They said she probably fled the country. Probably.

Later, Agent Cheever called me up to say they had arrested Hector Federinko, aka Aunt Agnes. They found him somewhere in Pennsylvania called Paradise. It was on that call that Agent Cheever also asked if I knew anything about tunnels that ran under the Pink Locker offices. Tunnels? Again, I had nothing.

School life readjusted to a different rhythm. I wasn't as busy. It felt OK to go at a slower pace, but I missed the work of the Pink Locker Society. It made me feel needed and smart. I learned a lot, including that I wasn't such a freak myself with all my many concerns. I also learned that everyone worries, at least a little, even Piper.

I missed getting thank-you letters from our…whatever they were… our customers, our clients, our friends? Who doesn't like a heap of praise? Not that I need applause all day long, but they always put a smile on my face. I kept one and only one of them by forwarding it to my home email account. I'm glad I did it, even though it was probably against the rules. But what did the rules matter now, given that criminals had been in charge? It said:

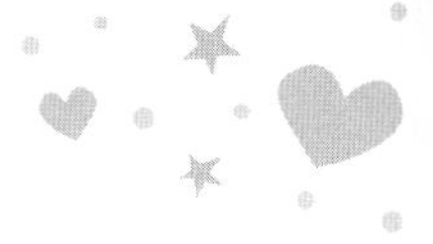

I thank you soooooooo much for creating this website. It makes me feel normal and special at the same time.

The Pink Locker Society did the same for me. And now, I just felt normal. Normal is OK, but it's a wee bit dull. That's why I was so glad when Agent Cheever called to say he wanted to drop off something for the three of us on Friday afternoon. In honor of whatever it was – a reward for aiding a federal investigation, maybe? – I invited Kate and Piper to my house for a sleepover.

"Viva la sleepovers!" Piper called out when I invited her on Thursday. She sometimes did this – took a phrase and tried to work it into every possible situation. One summer, she talked like a pirate from the time school let out until it started up again in August. But now she was on a Spanish kick. So instead of "Long live sleepovers!" or "Woo-hoo sleepovers!" Piper gave us "Viva la sleepovers!" I had to agree. May they never end!

We decided this sleepover should start right after school on Friday, so Piper and Kate walked home from school with me. The night stretched out ahead of us with good stuff planned: a movie, pizza, and then some joint decision-making about yearbook photos.

"Viva la FBI!" Piper yelled when the doorbell rang at my house.

Agent Cheever stood at my door with his new partner, Lucy Lamott. After the hellos and the introductions, she handed us a thick brown bag marked "EVIDENCE." Inside was our beloved pink laptop.

"All the data's been stripped," Agent Cheever said. "But I figured you girls might like it back."

"Lee here wanted it for his very own, but I told him no," Agent Lamott said.

"Yes, right. Tough guys like pink and all of that," he said, holding back a smile.

My mother narrowed her eyes a bit when she saw our reclaimed laptop, but then she said, "I guess it's all right as long as you use it for good."

"Viva la laptop!" Piper called out after the agents left and we were alone.

It was just a cold piece of plastic technology, but having the computer back sent us on a trip down memory lane.

"Remember our first meeting when Jem couldn't open the pink locker?" Piper said.

"And remember when Jem decided that Forrest needed a personal tour?" Kate said.

"Hey, does anyone remember that we actually did some good? People loved us. We had fans," I said.

"Let's turn it on," Piper said, "just for old time's sake."

"It's just a computer now. It's nice to have, but not that special anymore," I said.

"Let's see if there's anything left," Piper said, and spun the laptop toward her.

Meanwhile, between bites of pizza, Kate and I kept talking about all that had happened.

"If you could go back in time, would you do anything differently? Like maybe never step through the Pink Locker door?" Kate asked me.

"No, I think I'd still go. Well, I'd still go if you pulled me in."

"Oh, my gosh, remember the snacks? We're lucky they didn't poison us," Kate said.

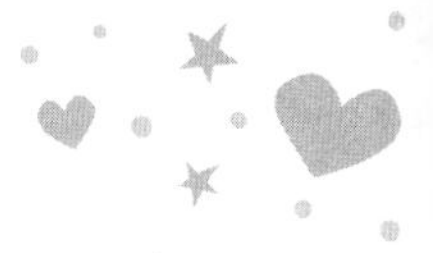

"Viva la snacks!" said Piper, pumping a fist in the air and then getting back to her clicking and clacking. We heard the laptop start humming, its internal fan started whirring, and simultaneously all three of our phones sprang to life. They chimed with that familiar tune – the opening bars of "Respect" – duh-nuh-nuh-duh-nuh-*nyah!*

We had mail – Pink Locker Society mail!

"It's probably just Piper cranking us," Kate said.

"Yeah, Pipes. That's cruel. You got us all excited," I said.

"Viva la email!" Piper said. "Look for yourselves."

She spun the laptop toward Kate and me and we saw it was true. Piper, the computer whiz, had somehow located our Pink Locker Society email and we had dozens of unread messages. Most of them came in more than a month ago before news started to trickle out that the site was down, apparently forever. We read each and every one.

My best friend stole my boyfriend. What do I do?

Can I go on vacation while I have my period?

People tease me because I don't wear makeup. What should I do?

I have a huge crush on my teacher. Help!

I do not have pretty feet. Should I wear sandals anyway?

I'm the shortest girl in my class and I'm sick of the nicknames. What should I do?

Everyone tells me I look fine, but I still feel fat. How can I lose weight?

On and on they went, a rainbow of woes. Each one represented a person's sincere question. Some were serious issues, others more minor, but each one mattered to someone.

"Gosh, this stinks that we can't answer any of them," Kate said.

"We've just abandoned them."

"Look how the number of emails trailed off in the last few weeks. They're forgetting about us," I said.

"Read this one," Piper said.

Hey, are you guys on vacation or something? I wrote twice and the website isn't working. It's kind of important. My parents are getting a divorce.

The more messages we read, the more our group mood took a plunge. We had started out all silly and happy. Just moments ago, Piper was shouting, "Viva la erasable pens!" and "Viva la flannel pajamas!" Now, at least 20 minutes had gone by without a "Viva la…" anything.

Instead, we kept murmuring at each other about how there was nothing we could do. What could we do? The Pink Locker Society was closed, by order of the FBI.

Or was it?

I looked at Kate. Kate looked at Piper and the two of them looked back at me.

"Nobody said we had to stop helping people," I said.

"Riiiiiight," Kate said, nodding slowly.

It was one of those cosmic friend moments. Silently, we were sharing the same thought – once again three flowers on the same stem. Piper stopped tapping on the keyboard. Kate held her triangle of pizza aloft on the palm of her hand. Sure, none of us knew exactly *how* we would do it. Not yet, anyway. But I knew what needed to be said. I, Jemma, jumped up on the couch and shouted it before Piper could beat me to it: **"Viva La Pink Locker Society!"**

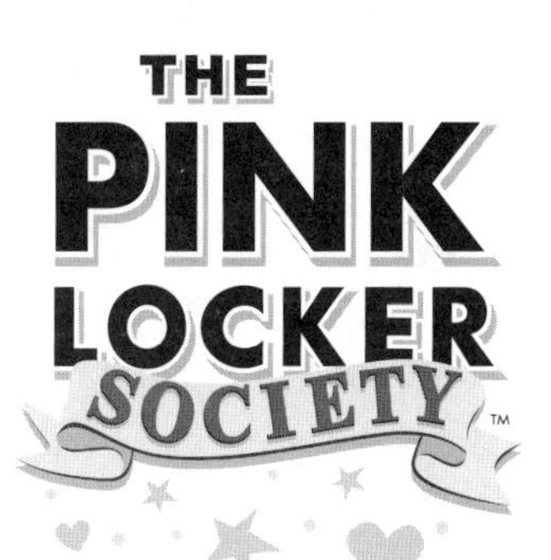

Viva La Pink Locker Society!

Now that you're a part of the club,
stay in the pink at

PinkLockerSociety.org

It's fun and free, so bring your BFF!
Ask questions and get answers.
Decorate your dream locker, make purses,
wish necklaces, and other creative
crafts. Try new recipes, give your
opinion, start a book club* and more!

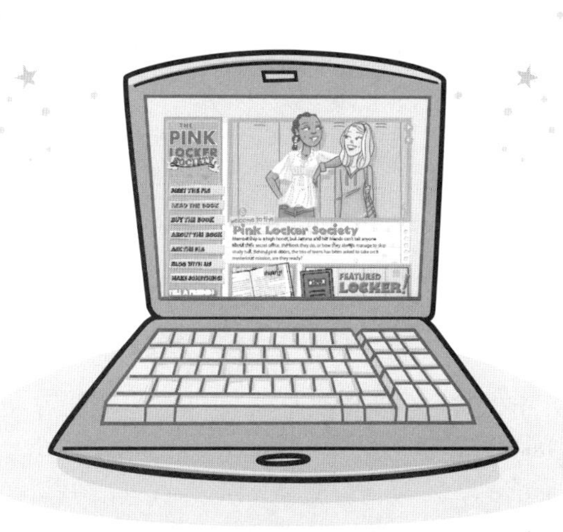

*See next page for tips on how to start a book club.

Start Your Own Book Club!

Everything is more fun with a friend, including reading a book. That's the whole idea behind book clubs. A group of friends read the same book, talk about it, and snack. What could be better than that?

Follow these steps to start your own book group:

1. Get the word out.
Round up 4-12 friends who like to read.

2. Schedule meeting dates.
It's important to space your meetings far enough apart so that members have enough time to read the books. Many clubs find that a monthly meeting works well, and that keeping it on the same day (such as the first Wednesday of every month) helps.

3. Pick a place.
Most clubs take turns meeting at someone's house, but they can really happen anywhere: after school in an empty classroom, at the public library, or even the local bookstore.

4. Plan for snacks.
What fun would a club be without snacks? For variety, ask two or three people to bring some munchies to each meeting.

5. Choose the books.
The most important thing! Decide how your group will pick the books. Some groups take turns letting each member choose. Others open it up to the group to decide.

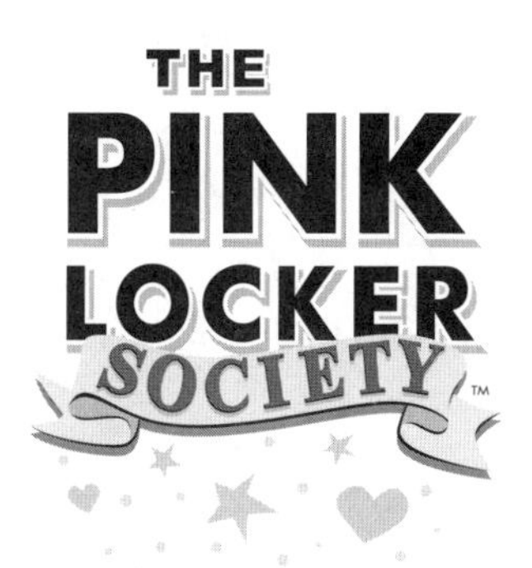

Questions & Answers

The PLS has answers! In this special bonus section, get their trusted advice on dozens of issues. And if you have a question of your own, visit pinklockersociety.org to submit it!

Dear PLS,
I have a problem in the boob department. One's bigger than the other. Help!
Lopsided

Dear Lopsided,
Relax! Girls grow a lot during these years and it's common for one breast to get ahead of the other. This usually evens out over time and you are probably the only one who has noticed this small imbalance in your bra. Speaking of bras, as you get older, if you are still a little uneven, you can always use padding on one side. Think pink!

Dear PLS,
Brown is the most boring color ever created. And it's the color of my boring hair. I want to dye it red, or possibly pink, but my mom says no. How old do you have to be to dye your hair?
Down With Brown

Dear D.W.B.,
Changing your hair is a fun way to experiment with your look, but the experts we asked said girls in middle school shouldn't mess with their hair color. Dyeing your hair means using chemicals on it. Some people report a burning or itching scalp – or even hair loss – after getting their hair dyed. But that aside, we think brown hair is nice. Is yours more golden brown or a darker brown like deep, dark chocolate? Instead of dyeing it, we'd recommend a new headband, haircut, or hairstyle. Think pink! (but not pink hair!)

Hey,
This is going to sound weird, but my boobs are ruining my life. They are ENOR-MOOSE boobs. Biggest in the school. What do I do?
Signed,
E.B.

Dear E.B.,
We hear you! Though lots of girls wish for bigger breasts, when you feel yours are too big, it is no fun. They always seem to get in the way. The

best approach is to manage them. Here are good steps to take:

1. Buy bras that fit you well. Go to a store that has someone who can measure and fit you for a bra. This may sound embarrassing, but it's worth it to get a bra that fits right and feels good. If there's no expert fitter, ask your mom, aunt, big sister, or a female friend to help. Also buy a sports bra so you feel comfortable when it's time for gym class or sports.

2. Choose clothes that work with your figure. A good bra will help you wear most any shirt you like, but if you're self-conscious, try not to wear shirts that are too tight or too revealing. You can do a quick check at home to see if your shirt is too revealing. Stand in front of a mirror and bend forward. Your shirt shouldn't open or gap too much.

3. Learn to handle gawkers. It's annoying to have people stare at your chest, but you never have to just put up with rude stares or comments. Tell a parent, teacher, or another adult if someone is bothering you in this way. You can ignore them and walk away but if you're feeling bold just tell the offending gawker: "Yo, my eyes are up here!" Think pink!

Dear PLS,
My grandma has breast cancer. I'm very worried about her. Why does this have to happen?
Grandma's Girl

Dear G.G.,
We're sorry to hear about your grandma. We love our grandmothers like no one else in the world. Even experts don't know exactly why someone gets breast cancer, but being older and having a history of it in the family can make a woman more likely to get it. Fortunately, doctors do know a lot about how to fight it. You can be helpful to your grandma by encouraging her during the treatments she is getting to fight the disease. You might consider wearing a pink ribbon or raising money for breast cancer research. A positive attitude can help your grandma – and you – during this time. Think pink!

Dear PLS,
OK, here's a problem for you. I accidentally tooted in class and everyone knows it was me. Now they're calling me Miss Farts A Lot!
Your friend,
Miss You Know What

Dear Miss Y.K.W.,
Oh, dear. That's not a nickname anyone would want. But the truth is that everyone passes gas because everyone digests food. Of course, we'd rather not do it in public, but it happens. If you find yourself feeling gassy again, go to the bathroom or find an out-of-the-way spot. Our guess is that your nickname will eventually fade away. If someone teases you about it in the meantime, remind him or her that everybody toots! Think pink!

Dear PLS,
Can I swim when I have my period? If so, won't people see the pad in my bathing suit?
Signed,
Super Swimmer

Dear S.S.,
Yes, you can swim when you have your period. Getting exercise is fun and healthy, so you don't want to avoid something you love. But a girl should wear a tampon to swim. Like a pad, a tampon absorbs the menstrual flow but it does so from inside the vagina. A tampon is made of absorbent material that is pressed into a cylinder shape. Learning to insert a tampon takes a little practice, but just relax and be patient. Talk to your mom, sister, or someone else who has experience using tampons. Read the directions in the package and remember to change it every 4 to 6 hours. Think pink!

Dear PLS,
My backpack is very heavy. It's like carrying rocks to school every day. How can I get my teachers to give me less homework?
Signed,
Weighed Down

Dear W.D.,
This one was a toughie. After about two seconds of discussion, we realized that teachers were not going to ease up on the homework. So the only other solution is to carry less weight and carry it in a way that doesn't hurt your back. We hope these tips lighten your load!

1. Take stock of what's in your backpack and figure out if you need every item and book in there. We sometimes find balled up sweatshirts, pieces of long-ago lunches, and lots of pennies and nickles swimming in the depths of our backpacks.

2. Use both shoulder straps. We have been guilty of just using one, but two balances the load so we're not afraid to use both.

3. Do wheelies! Consider a rolling backpack so you can roll it instead of haul it on your back. Think pink!

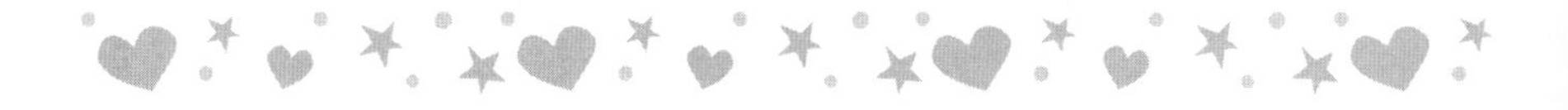

Dear PLS,
I know this is a website for girls, but I'm a guy. Here's my question: All the guys I know like the same girl. It makes me mad because I've liked her the longest. How can I tell those other guys to back off?
Signed,
A Guy

Dear A.G.,

We're happy to know that guys like our website, too. Everyone is welcome here! But back to your question. It stinks when too many people – especially friends – like the same person. In some ways, it's like in soccer or basketball when everyone is fighting for the ball. Hey, that's mine! Give it here! But a girl (or a guy) isn't a piece of sporting equipment. People aren't property, so there's no sense telling other boys they shouldn't like "your" girl. But you can tell this girl that you like her and see what happens. Even though you liked her first, it's up to her to decide whom she likes. Maybe she likes you, too. But be kind if she just wants to be friends. Think pink (or blue)!

About the Author

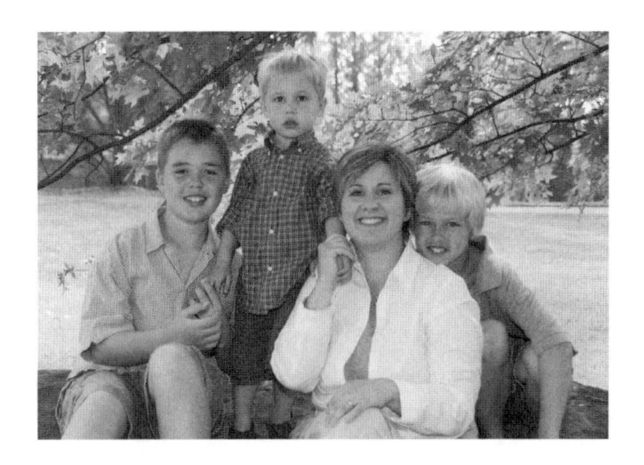

Debra Moffitt is the kids' editor of KidsHealth.org – the #1 website for health information written just for kids. In her role, Moffitt receives email from thousands of tweens – most of them girls. They write in with questions about their changing bodies and (sometimes urgent) requests for advice in dealing with the ups and downs of middle school life. Thanks to their daily inquiries and shared stories, *The Pink Locker Society* was born.

Before joining KidsHealth in 2002, Moffitt was a newspaper reporter and an online journalist. She received a fellowship in fiction writing in 2006 from the Delaware Division of the Arts. Her nonfiction writing has appeared in the *Washington Post* and the *Miami Herald*. Moffitt was also the editor of *Fit Kids*, a KidsHealth book for parents published in 2004 by Dorling Kindersley. Moffitt lives in Delaware with her husband and three sons, ages 12, 11, and 3.

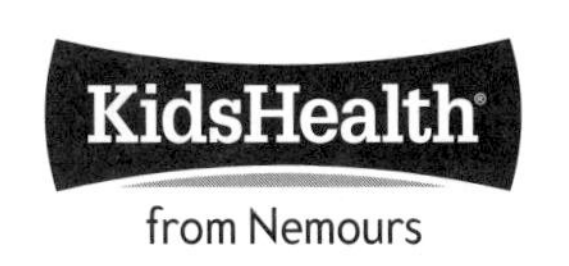

Every year more than 170 million families, educators, health professionals, and media turn to KidsHealth.org, making it the #1 most-visited website devoted to children's health. KidsHealth is physician-led, providing doctor-approved health information about the physical, emotional, and behavioral health of children – from before birth through adolescence. KidsHealth.org features three distinct sections – for parents, for kids, and for teens – each with its own tone and age-appropriate topics.

KidsHealth is known for its engaging, family-friendly information. Recent accolades include the 2008 Parents' Choice Gold Award for Best Website for Kids and Webby Awards for both the Best Family/Parenting Website and Best Health Website. KidsHealth was also named one of the "50 Coolest Websites" by *TIME*.

KidsHealth comes from The Nemours Center for Children's Health Media. The Center creates print, online, and video content about a wide range of children's health topics. KidsHealth also works with health providers, insurers, and corporations to provide family-friendly health information and materials specifically for parents, kids, and teens. KidsHealth is part of Nemours, one of the largest nonprofit organizations devoted to children's health and development.